PRAISE

"Jenny has done a tremendous job in bringing back awareness to a critically important subject – how gluten threatens our health. No, the problem never went away. But avoiding gluten, although fundamentally important for health, has become yet another inconvenient truth. Jenny provides the latest science confirming gluten's role in so many modern-day maladies and provides a cogent approach to navigating a healthful gluten-free life."

—David Perlmutter, MD,
and #1 *New York Times* bestselling
author of *Grain Brain* and *Brain Maker*

"Jenny not only makes a compelling case for why gluten is hurting so many people, but also she shows us exactly what we need to do to get it out of our lives for good. But Jenny doesn't stop there. She goes where few books about celiac disease have gone before by showing us how she healed her body beyond the gluten-free diet, and how she put her celiac disease into remission and reclaimed her health once and for all."

—Jill C. Carnahan,
MD ABIHM, ABIoM, IFMCP and
Medical Director of Flatiron Functional Medicine

"Jenny is the patient expert when it comes to healing celiac disease and gluten sensitivity with good nutrition. Her astute knowledge makes breaking up with gluten and going gluten free much less daunting."

—Elana Amsterdam
New York Times bestselling author of
The Gluten-Free Almond Flour Cookbook
and founder of *Elana's Pantry*

"I develop gluten-free recipes for a living, motivated by a desire to cater to my son's gluten-free diet, to ensure that his food is at least as good, if not better, than everyone else's. But the moment we leave the house, I'm out of my depth. Jenny's book will help you understand your diagnosis, advocate for yourself and your health, and deal with the intense emotions that are unavoidable along the way. Jenny truly understands what it means to live a healthy, gluten-free lifestyle that goes well beyond breaking things off with gluten."

—Nicole Hunn,
founder and author of
Gluten Free on a Shoestring

"Jenny is a tireless advocate for the celiac disease and broader gluten-free community. Her debut book is an accessible entrée for the newly gluten free – equal parts personal journey, educational resource, and lifestyle guide."

—Kelli and Pete Bronski,
co-founders of No Gluten, No Problem,
and co-authors of *No Gluten, No Problem Pizza*
and *Artisanal Gluten-Free Cooking*

"In *Dear Gluten, It's Not Me, It's You*, Jenny provides a clear road map on how to make the split with gluten and begin the long healing process from the damage it causes to sensitive individuals. Her practical tips and authentic voice offer readers guidance, assurance, and hope when transitioning to a gluten-free lifestyle."

—Scott Adams, CEO of Celiac.com

"Jenny provides a real-life perspective on what it's like to live a gluten-free lifestyle. Her blueprint for improving gut health and healing your entire body is comprehensive and goes beyond just eating gluten-free foods. Jenny's personal story is one so many of us can relate to and her lovely way of helping us heal will benefit everyone dealing with health challenges. I highly encourage everyone that is struggling with their health to read this book and finally start to heal your whole body."

—Jen Cafferty, founder and
CEO of The Nourished Group

"Jenny is a force in the gluten-free community. She has been advocating on healthy lifestyle and choices, not just eating gluten free. Removing gluten from your life is often difficult and filled with emotions. Jenny helps you to work through those emotions in this amazing book. With her blueprint you can now take the next steps to healing your body. Anyone with a gluten intolerance needs this book to start on their path to healing."

—Jennifer Bigler,
founder of Living Freely Gluten Free and
author of *101 Incredible Gluten-Free Recipes*

"The Hollywood gluten-free fad left a perception about the diet that is often misunderstood. Jenny clears things up beautifully with, "*Dear Gluten, It's Not Me, It's You*". Finally, a fresh and humanistic perspective on the gluten-free diet with relevant and current information."

—Josh Schieffer, author of *Gluten-Free Buyers Guide*

DEAR GLUTEN

IT'S NOT ME, IT'S YOU

*How to survive without gluten and
restore your health from celiac disease or
gluten sensitivity*

JENNY LEVINE FINKE

Certified Integrative Nutrition Coach

DEAR GLUTEN, IT'S NOT ME, IT'S YOU
How to Survive Without Gluten and Restore Your Health
from Celiac Disease or Gluten Sensitivity
By JENNY LEVINE FINKE
1. HEA039090 2. HEA039010 3. HEA017000
ISBN: 978-1-949642-43-8
EBOOK: 978-1-949642-44-5

Cover design by LEWIS AGRELL

Printed in the United States of America

Authority Publishing
11230 Gold Express Dr. #310-413
Gold River, CA 95670
800-877-1097
www.AuthorityPublishing.com

DISCLAIMERS

Information in this book should not be treated as a substitute for professional assistance from trained medical, health, and wellness professionals. Readers should discuss any changes to their diets, medications, supplements, treatments, diagnosis, and physical activities with their doctor before taking any action as a result of information from this book.

The reader acknowledges that implementation of any diet or activity is at the sole discretion of the reader's choice and initiative, and the reader assumes full responsibility for his or her understanding, interpretations, and actions as a result. The author of this book assumes no responsibility for the actions of the reader. This book should solely be used to elicit discussion with the reader's doctor and/or trained healthcare professionals.

The author has done her best to provide accurate information in this book, and when necessary, provide a source for information shared. The author, however, does not guarantee the accuracy of any details in this book, and each reader should do his or her due diligence on any claim or information presented.

The author of this book has worked in paid collaboration with several of the brands mentioned in this book. No compensation has been received for inclusion of any brand in this book.

DEDICATION

To every gluten-free person who has struggled, been dismissed, doubted, or made to feel less than, this book is for you.

"You are imperfect, you are wired for struggle, but you are worthy of love and belonging."

- Brené Brown

CONTENTS

PART I: THE BREAKUP

PART II: THE HEALING

PART III: THE RECIPES

PREFACE

Have you ever done something a certain way your whole life and then one day, woken up and realized you've been doing it all wrong?

This is how I felt when I learned I had celiac disease. I had the sudden realization that I had been eating wrong my entire life. Everything I *thought* I knew about food, nutrition, and what was and wasn't good for me was wrong. Dead wrong.

On my journey to re-learn how to eat, I discovered Dr. Tom O'Bryan, a world-renowned expert in gluten-related disorders. I've followed Dr. O'Bryan's work for many years, listening to all his podcast interviews and devouring his books and lectures. His words speak to me. They make sense. He helped me realize how many people are suffering in this world due to gluten.

This is why I asked Dr. O'Bryan to write the Foreword of my book. He has shaped my thinking like none other. He has taught me that gluten is the source of pain for so many people, that you don't have to have a celiac disease diagnosis to know gluten is no good for you, and that gluten can be a precursor to autoimmune disease and other serious disorders.

This book is dedicated to the entire gluten-free community. Whether you eat gluten free because you have celiac disease, a wheat allergy, gluten sensitivity, an autoimmune disease, or you simply feel better without gluten (no judgment here!), you will always have a place at my gluten-free table. I hope to make you feel loved, respected, and understood in the pages of this book.

FOREWORD

LOVING KINDNESS IN THE TRENCHES

In the summer of 1984, the Australian gastroenterologist Barry Marshall had claimed, "Sometimes, I believe ulcers can be caused by a bacteria." He was labeled a "nutcase" because everyone knew that ulcers were caused by too much hydrochloric acid produced in the stomach, and that you had to take antacids to calm down ulcers.

So what did he do? He took some bacteria from a petri dish, had them mixed with lukewarm beef extract – the normal nutrient solution for bacteria in the lab – and filled a little more than one cup into a beaker. Then he downed it without complaining. He drank a beaker of bacteria and waited to see what would happen.

Three days later, Marshall felt nauseated and his mother told him he had bad breath. Next he started vomiting. Gastroscopy confirmed ulcers in his stomach. But he still waited a few days before taking the antibiotics that were supposed to kill the bacteria in his stomach. A follow-up gastroscopy confirmed the ulcers were gone and clarified his diagnosis: His ulcers were caused by the bacteria, which when eliminated, immediately allowed the stomach to heal.

He didn't care that everyone thought he was wrong, and that ulcers were caused by too much acid. Period. End of story. Well, "everyone" was wrong. The World Health Organization sent a message to every medical society in the world about Dr. Marshall's concept that *Helicobacter pylori* (*H. pylori*), sometimes, is the cause of ulcers. Why did they do that? Because if you identify an *H.*

pylori infection with heartburn, acute gastritis (an inflammation of the stomach), and eradicate it, you also eliminate the most common cause of the #1 cancer in the world at the time, stomach cancer. Yes, *H. pylori* is the primary trigger to stomach cancer.

It took Dr. Marshall, holding his own against every peer, every doctor who heard of his theory and thought he was a "nutcase," to bring to the world the (now) unquestionable fact that *H. pylori* can be a problem.

For his courage, Dr. Marshall and his long-time research partner, Dr. Robin Warren, 21 years later, in 2005, won the Nobel Prize in Physiology or Medicine. And the quote from the Nobel Committee for these two men? Drs. Barry Marshall and Robin Warren, "Who with tenacity and a prepared mind, challenged prevailing dogma."

Because Drs. Marshall and Warren stood their ground, millions are better today. Stomach cancer is no longer the #1 cancer in the world. People are diagnosed much sooner with an *H. pylori* infection and it's taken care of and never has a chance to progress to stomach cancer. They stood their ground, and so does Jenny Levine Finke. No one, absolutely no one, can argue with her (or with me for that matter) that for some people, gluten, and any form of wheat, can be a problem manifesting between a little ache and pain to life-threatening diseases. Her book is a road map of working your way through the trenches, through tenacity, and preparing your own mind so you win your own Nobel Prize in the best health of your life.

She does an excellent job laying out her story and experiences that stem from years of suffering, and explains why, despite everything, doctors and the general population still resist – and even dismiss – the gluten-free diet. Why is there so much resistance? Because almost everyone thinks of bread as the "staff of life." We've all grown up feasting at the table of wheat at most meals. From toast to sandwiches to pasta, it is the most common food eaten in the world today.[1]

Many of us grew up with the phrase, "Give us this day our daily bread…"

But as the journal *Frontiers in Neuroscience* wrote on the first page of its 2016 article titled *Bread and Other Edible Agents of Mental Disease*, "Give us this day our daily bread (. . .) but deliver us from evil." -Matthew 6:11, 13.[2]

Yes, bread can fuel mental diseases like depression, anxiety, schizophrenia, and Alzheimer's. It also can fuel chronic fatigue, hormone imbalances, psoriasis, thyroid autoimmune disease, acne, MS, lupus, or... the list goes on and on. That's why there are more than 23,000 studies on wheat and different diseases. It just depends on your genetic vulnerability, the weak link in your chain, as to where it will manifest. Manifest it will, regardless if it's at age two, 22, or 92. Chronic disease is fueled by inflammation. The majority of inflammation is fueled by what's on the end of your fork... and wheat is the most common food sensitivity when tested for.

In *Dear Gluten: It's Not Me, It's You*, Jenny does an excellent job of writing from the trenches. She writes what it's like to get out of the trenches and to thrive (food wise) more than ever before. With topics like how to eat at a buffet, dining while traveling, medications and beauty products, handling accidental exposures, how to read menus, and what questions to ask, she's already gone through the mud in the trenches, fallen on her face, and picked herself right back up again. If you think the topic of medications and beauty products is not of interest? Look up this study of wheat-dependent exercise-induced anaphylaxis (WDEIA), where healthy athletes went into asthmatic attacks while exercising because of a soap they had used that had wheat in it.[3] [4]

When you listen to the stories of world class athletes and Olympians who were pushing through their pains and fatigues for years, and then go gluten free and feel like new people, and go on to win Olympic gold and break world records because gluten is no longer holding them back, you realize that you never would have guessed that this most-common food could be such a trigger.

Perhaps the greatest gift of Jenny's book is her remarkable realization that, "I wish I had been kinder to myself back then, realizing that I was just at the start line of a very long marathon that would continue for the rest of my life. The first hours, days, and weeks are the hardest. I kept reminding myself, this too shall pass."

She probably doesn't know it, but Jenny is expressing an ancient Tibetan theme called Maitri. Loosely translated, it means, "Loving-kindness and an unconditional friendship with one's self."

My prayer for you with this outstanding roadmap of a book is that you operate with loving-kindness, too, as you find your way out of the trenches.

Dr. Tom O'Bryan, DC, CCN, DACBN, CFMP

Dr. O'Bryan is the author of *The Autoimmune Fix: How to Stop the Hidden Autoimmune Damage that Keeps You Sick, Fat, and Tired*, and *You Can Fix Your Brain: Just 1 Hour a Week to the Best Memory, Productivity, and Sleep You've Ever Had*. Find him at www.theDr.com.

INTRODUCTION

"Medicine is not only a science; it is also an art. It does not consist of compounding pills and plasters; it deals with the very processes of life, which must be understood before they may be guided."

- Paracelsus, 16th century physician, alchemist, theologian and philosopher

Breaking up is hard to do. I ate gluten for 34 years of my life, and I enjoyed every bite of bread, pasta, and cake I could get my hands on. Then I had to give it up cold turkey after my doctor diagnosed me with celiac disease. I had to change my relationship status with gluten from "in a relationship" to "it's complicated." My love affair with gluten ended suddenly and abruptly.

Giving up a food group I had loved so dearly for my entire life was extremely difficult. While I was relieved to know the root cause of my painful bloating and embarrassing gas, I deeply mourned the loss of gluten and the easy-breezy life I once had with gluten by my side.

Like many people who struggle with a difficult breakup, I turned to comfort food. What in the world was I supposed to eat now? A big bowl of pasta sounded good, as did a slice of sourdough bread. But I couldn't turn to those comfort foods anymore; they are, after all, the exact foods that got me into this mess in the first place. A hard-boiled egg, while naturally gluten free, is hardly comfort food, nor is kale.

It was time to make sense of my new life without gluten. It was time to get back into the "dating" game and forge ahead with a new (and hopefully) better relationship with food. I read every book I could find. I Googled every question I had. I even enrolled in the Institute for Integrative Nutrition, where I became a certified integrative nutrition health coach, on my quest to understand what was going on inside of me. I removed every crumb of gluten from my life, yet I was only marginally better. I remained bloated and gassy; and on top of it all, I couldn't stop thinking about my ex. Was there more to this gluten-free diet than meets the eye?

WHY I WROTE THIS BOOK

This book is a direct result of my discovering that breaking up with gluten is hard yet a necessary step to reclaiming one's health. I want to share current research on why gluten disorders are on the rise, why gluten is the source of disease for so many people, why there is a huge uptick in diagnosed gluten disorders today, and what readers need to do to heal their bodies and restore their health sans gluten. I focus on healing and restoring whole-body health.

As I began thinking about what I wanted this book to look like, I came across an adorable shirt from CeliacCutie™ that says, "*Dear Gluten, We are never, ever getting back together.*" I love the play on words from the famous Taylor Swift song with the same name (minus the "Dear Gluten" part). This shirt captured my experience perfectly because being diagnosed with a gluten disorder feels like a bad, permanent, *we are never getting back together* kind of affair.

The idea of *breaking up* with gluten stuck with me for a long time, and I had this disquieting sentiment that I needed to put into words how I was feeling. I wrote a blog post titled "The Emotional Burden of the Gluten-Free Diet," where I talked about the emotional aspects that came along with my split with gluten. The article resonated with so many people and inspired me to explore this topic further. As I reflected on my eight-year gluten-free journey, it was evident that I had gone through all the *feelings* involved with breaking up with a long-time boyfriend – relief, shock, frustration, physical and emotional distress, isolation, grief, and even anger and resentment until I finally made peace with my fate and found a way to turn proverbial lemons into lemonade.

Dear Gluten, It's Not Me, It's You is my journey to understand the factors that led to my breakup with gluten, how I let go of my bad boy ex, and my journey to heal my body and reconcile my life without gluten in it.

There is so much information floating around out there, and it's hard to know whom to believe. I hope this book will help you make sense of it all so you can figure out what works for you and you alone. I'm not a doctor or scientist; rather, I'm someone who lives this way of life day in and day out. I'm someone who has struggled to figure out how to bake gluten-free bread, someone who has cried in the bathroom of a restaurant because the waiter messed up my order, and someone who has worked hard to heal her body from the ravages of celiac disease, all with a little grace and a whole lot of grit.

Like all breakups, breaking up with gluten can be challenging, emotional, and painful. I hope you find solace in knowing you are not alone, and that this book serves as a beacon of light guiding you through your journey to become *free from* gluten's power over you.

WHOM IS THIS BOOK FOR?

Having picked up this book, you are likely questioning your relationship status with gluten. You may have had a swift breakup with gluten after receiving a celiac disease or gluten sensitivity diagnosis. (Please note that I use the terms gluten sensitivity and gluten intolerance interchangeably throughout this book.)

Or perhaps you haven't left gluten yet, but you either intuitively know it's *not good* for you and you've struggled to let gluten go, or you've wondered if a gluten-free diet will help you manage your *fill-in-the-blank* health ailment.

This book is also for you if you're avoiding gluten for any reason and wonder if the effort needed to stay gluten free is worth it. Because it takes drastic measures to implement and stay on a gluten-free diet, you might be asking yourself, "Is gluten *really* damaging my body?" "Is it gluten that is making and keeping me sick?" "Will eating even a little gluten have *dire* effects on my health?" If you've struggled to understand how gluten is in the wrong, I will help you see why even a one-night stand with this bad boy is just not worth it.

Honestly, whatever your relationship status with gluten, this book is for you. I will help you understand how gluten is negatively impacting your life and why breaking up with something you've loved for so long might just be the best decision you will ever make (and how it might even save your life!). I think we can all agree that sometimes you have to let go of something you love even if it's hard or unpopular to do.

What You'll Find

Here is what you will find in this book:

Part I: The Breakup: I'll help you see gluten's true colors. It won't take long for you to understand why gluten is the source of woe in your life. Understanding why gluten is up to no good will help you feel confident breaking up with the damaging protein once and for all. I'll also show you how to consciously uncouple with gluten.

Part II: The Healing: It takes time to heal physically, emotionally, and spiritually when breaking up with gluten. You may have shown gluten the door, but have you taken time to heal the scars left behind from your torrid love affair? Unfortunately, most doctors don't help you with the healing part. They tell you to avoid gluten and then send you on your merry way. They don't tell you how to *heal* your body, mind, and soul from the damage left behind from gluten's reign of terror. I'll give you tips you can implement right now to help you heal your insides, restore your health, and reclaim your life. Skip ahead to this section if you're suffering from chronic health issues despite eating gluten free.

Part III: The Recipes: I'll show you how to recreate many of your favorite recipes without gluten as well as how to create new and delicious meals for you and your family, all with a focus on healing your body via the power of food.

Thank you for inviting me to be your guide on your gluten-free journey. I hope the wisdom from my formerly-broken-now-healed body will help make your split with gluten a little easier.

Sincerely,
Jenny

PART I

THE BREAKUP

DEAR GLUTEN LETTER

Dear Gluten:

This isn't going to be easy, so I'm just going to come out and say it: It's time for us to break up. I cannot "be" with you anymore.

This has been a gut-wrenching decision for me. I desperately want to be healthy and happy again, and the only path forward for me is without you.

There were many times we loafed around together. I loved the way you smelled and tasted. You comforted me in times of sadness. You were always there for me when I needed you most. I craved you then, and I know I will crave you in the future. But, I must resist you more than ever now that I know we are not meant to be.

You look all innocent and dough-eyed, but the truth is you're slowly tearing away the lining of my gut. You're making and keeping me sick. We are fundamentally incompatible.

I have put a lot of thought into my decision. I wish I could say I'd like to remain friends, but the truth is our relationship must end. You are hurting me, and even an occasional rendezvous with you makes me sick to my stomach, literally.

We must go our separate ways, forever. Please don't try to talk me out of this. My decision is final.

Farewell, Gluten.
Jenny

CHAPTER 1
BREAKING UP IS HARD TO DO

"You may not control all the events that happen to you, but you can decide not to be reduced by them."

–Maya Angelou

Breaking up is hard to do. In 2012, I went through one of the hardest breakups of my life when I split with gluten.

I was sitting in my car in the airport parking lot eating a Subway® sandwich, sipping on a Diet Coke®, and checking emails on my phone as I waited for my parent's flight to land. My phone rang; it was my doctor.

To give you a little background, I had visited my doctor the prior week for my annual checkup. I told her I was experiencing painful, chronic bloating and really annoying gas, especially at night. I asked her to prescribe or recommend a gas medication to help me. She instead suggested we first run "some tests" as she said my symptoms didn't sound "normal" to her. I didn't even think to ask her what tests; I just went with it. I was anxious to get this chronic bloating and gas discomfort under control.

When my doctor's number popped up on my phone a week later, I thought nothing of it. I figured she was going to tell me everything was fine and that she would finally succumb to prescribing me that gas medication I had requested so I could relieve my chronic symptoms. However, the reason she called was to tell me that the tests revealed that I had celiac disease. I didn't see it coming. Gluten and I had had a wonderful relationship for 34 years; and now, in a matter of seconds, our relationship turned from *ignorance is bliss* to *what the heck just happened!* I was shocked.

My doctor went on to say that I should no longer eat gluten. She explained that gluten is a protein found mainly in wheat, barley, and rye; it is used to make foods like bread, pizza, and pasta – the exact three foods I loved dearly. The whole conversation is a blur now, but I remember listening intently to what she said as I held back the waterworks pooling in my eyes.

I recall asking her if I should stop eating gluten immediately, as in "right now," and she said yes. She suggested I talk with a nutrition professional to help me figure it all out.

A large lump began to form in my throat, so I thanked her for her time and hung up. I tossed the remaining sandwich in the nearby trashcan and proceeded with my day. My heart was broken. It felt like it had been stabbed with a thousand knives. Gluten and I were no longer meant to be, and now I had to figure out why this happened and what to do going forward. While I had no idea at the time how difficult the journey would be, I did know that the only way *to* was *through*. I would have to learn to accept my fate and figure out how to live my life without gluten in it.

Unfortunately, I'm not the only person suddenly forced to end a relationship with gluten. Three million people in the United States struggle with celiac disease today, and 18 million people in the U.S. suffer from gluten sensitivity. Although one in 100 people have celiac disease worldwide, only 20 percent of those with the disorder actually know they have it. If an immediate family member has celiac disease, the risk of having celiac disease increases to 1 in 10.[5]

WHAT IS CELIAC DISEASE?

Celiac disease, named for the Greek word "koilakos," which means abdominal, is an autoimmune disease in which your body attacks the healthy tissue that lines your small intestine every time you eat gluten. The constant attack slowly deteriorates the delicate, paper-thin lining of your gut, makes the proper digestion of your food and absorption of the food's nutrients near-impossible, and wreaks havoc throughout your entire body. If you have celiac disease, every time you eat gluten, your white blood cells produce antibodies that attack the healthy tissue lining the small intestine. This results in chronic damage to the intestinal mucosa or the inner wall of the small intestine.

The small intestine is a 20-25-foot-long tube lined with microvilli. Microvilli are follicles that protrude from the small intestine and look a lot like fingers. They serve an essential role in your digestive system. They soak up nutrients from food and help your body distribute those nutrients where they need to be to keep you healthy. If you have celiac disease, your microvilli are completely worn down and look more like a flat surface than fingers. When the microvilli are destroyed, the small intestine no longer has the ability to fully absorb nutrients from food. This is why most people with celiac disease suffer from some sort of nutritional deficiency such as anemia, low-blood sugar bouts, Vitamin B deficiency, and/or osteoporosis.

Normal villi

Villous atrophy

Normal mucosa
HEALTHY

Damaged mucosa
CELIAC DISEASE

WHAT CAUSES CELIAC DISEASE?

Researchers say three factors must be present in order for celiac disease to come to life.[6] First, you must have one of the celiac genes, which are HLA-DQ2 or HLA-DQ8. According to the Celiac Disease Center at the University of Chicago, one-third of the U.S. population carries one of the genes for celiac disease, yet only about three to five percent of those with either gene will eventually develop the disease.[7] This means that genes alone do not determine whether or not you will get celiac disease.

In addition to having one of the two celiac disease genes, you also must be consuming gluten, the trigger food. Celiac disease is the only autoimmune disease in which the trigger (gluten) is known.[8] Unfortunately, if you have other autoimmune conditions such as Crohn's, MS, Hashimoto's thyroiditis, or any of the hundreds of classified autoimmune diseases known to researchers, the "trigger" is still a mystery. This is why many researchers are zeroed in on studying celiac disease as it may aid in identifying the "trigger" or root cause of other autoimmune diseases.

Additionally, for the celiac disease genes to turn on or activate, you must experience intestinal permeability or leaky gut. When your gut is damaged, undigested proteins from the foods you eat "leak" into your bloodstream and wreak havoc at different sites in your body depending on where you are genetically most vulnerable. That's why celiac disease symptoms can seemingly turn on at any time, and why they go beyond bloating and diarrhea to include common but lesser known symptoms such as skin disorders, low bone density, failure to thrive, and migraines.

Researchers at New York University School of Medicine found the first measurable tie between celiac disease and environmental exposure to toxic chemicals found in pesticides, nonstick cookware, and flame retardants,[9] although environmental toxins have long been linked to inflammation and the development of autoimmune diseases. When researchers examined the levels of these toxins in the blood samples of 88 children and young adults, they found that the subjects with high blood levels of pesticide and pesticide-related chemicals called dichlorodiphenyldichloroeth-ylenes (DDEs) were twice as likely to be diagnosed with celiac disease. While the research is new, and the sample size small, it's worth noting that what we put in our bodies, even in passing, can affect gene expression.

We also know that celiac disease can appear at any age. The majority of people with celiac disease are diagnosed later in life, with a mean age of diagnosis at 46 years old. Of those newly diagnosed, 20 percent are over the age of 60. While the reason for adult-onset celiac disease can differ depending on which researcher you ask, many experts agree that some sort of gastro-intestinal episode, viral infection, trauma, surgery, pregnancy, or even overwhelming lifestyle stressors, along with a constant drip of gluten in the system, can serve as triggers that turn on the celiac disease genes later in life.[10] [11]

WHAT IS NON-CELIAC GLUTEN SENSITIVITY?

Non-celiac gluten (or wheat) sensitivity (NCGS or NCWS) – referred to as "gluten sensitivity" or "gluten intolerance" – is only just starting to be recognized as a real medical disorder. Unfortunately, there is still a lot of confusing information about how to classify, diagnose, and treat gluten sensitivity.

When someone is sensitive to gluten, it means they experience some sort of inflammatory response every time they consume gluten. Unlike people with celiac disease who clearly have a damaged intestine and experience total villous atrophy, people with gluten sensitivity may have normal looking and functioning villi. People with gluten sensitivity also do not develop antibodies to gluten like those with celiac disease.

While gluten sensitivity is considered a gluten disorder, it is not classified as an autoimmune disease, at least at this time. However, gluten sensitivity, if untreated, can be just as serious, and sometimes even more serious than celiac disease. People with gluten sensitivity often develop and experience the same symp-toms as those with celiac disease when exposed to gluten. If the disorder is unmanaged, it can lead to the same chronic symptoms and eventual damaging diseases as celiac disease.

Like celiac disease, gluten sensitivity is a permanent condition. Once you have it, you always have it, even if you heal. Dr. Tom O'Bryan, the author of *The Autoimmune Fix* and thought-leader on non-celiac gluten sensitivity (who wrote the Foreword of this book), says your body produces memory B cells to wheat (similar to what you produce when you receive a vaccination). These cells remember that they don't like wheat, and this is why your sensitivity to wheat is permanent.[12]

Unfortunately, gluten sensitivity is neither widely understood nor accepted by many doctors and patients. This is unfortunate for many reasons because it's a real disorder negatively impacting millions of people. If you suffer from gluten sensitivity, one study published in *Clinical Gastroenterology and Hepatology* might give you some comfort in knowing you are doing the right thing by breaking things off with gluten. Researchers performed a randomized, double-blind, placebo-controlled, crossover trial to determine the effect of low doses of gluten in people with suspected gluten sensitivity. Researchers enrolled 61 adults in the study who believed gluten was to blame for their intestinal and extraintestinal symptoms. None of them had tested positive for celiac disease or wheat allergy. Half of the participants were given a capsule of gluten and the other half were given a capsule of rice starch (placebo). After one week, the participants were given the reverse capsule. Researchers found those taking the gluten capsule experienced "significantly more severe" symptoms including but not limited to abdominal bloating and pain, foggy mind, depression, and/or mouth ulcers, when compared to the subjects taking the placebo.[13]

Regardless, both celiac disease and non-celiac gluten sensitivity are lifelong afflictions with no cure; you cannot get rid of or grow out of either disorder. However, the good news is you can put your symptoms into remission. Remission means you have no signs or symptoms of either disorder. It doesn't mean you're cured or no longer have celiac disease or gluten sensitivity; rather, it means that because you are no longer eating gluten, a blood test or biopsy can no longer detect celiac disease in your body and you will not experience the painful and annoying symptoms caused by either disorder. Should you begin eating gluten again, your symptoms will resurface, often with a vengeance, and the damage will reemerge.

GLUTEN CAUSES INFLAMMATION IN ALL HUMANS

Even if you don't have celiac disease or gluten sensitivity, the fact is that gluten is up to no good inside your body. One of the leading celiac disease researchers in the world, Dr. Alessio Fasano, along with a team of researchers, found that a peptide in wheat (gliadin) induces intestinal permeability (leaky gut) in all individuals whether or not they have celiac disease.[14] Let that sink in for a minute. Gluten causes inflammation of the gut in *all* who consume it, and it's widely accepted that inflammation is a precursor to a slew of degenerative conditions.

In this study published in *Nutrients* in 2015, researchers examined four strains of wheat, including two hybrid strains commonly used in the U.S. and two ancient strains. They divided test subjects into four subsets:

(1) individuals recently diagnosed with celiac
(2) people with celiac disease on a gluten-free diet for at least one year
(3) people with non-celiac gluten sensitivity
(4) people who had no problem eating gluten

Researchers found that all four groups experienced intestinal permeability when exposed to gliadin, a protein found in wheat. In other words, researchers found hard evidence that gluten activates the genes for intestinal permeability in all who eat it, not just in people with celiac disease or gluten sensitivity.[15]

When you eat gluten time and time again, you begin to chip away at the health of your intestinal lining. Most of the time your intestinal lining will repair itself; however, if you are predisposed to celiac disease or have gluten sensitivity, your gut may become damaged to the point where it is no longer able to restore and heal itself. This results in intestinal permeability or leaky gut, and it's where your health may start to go awry.

In fact, Dr. O'Bryan says in *The Autoimmune Fix* that when your gut becomes leaky, improperly digested bits of food particles "leak" into your bloodstream where they wreak havoc at different weak or genetically vulnerable spots in your body. If your vulnerable spot is your thyroid, you'll likely experience thyroid dysfunction. If your vulnerable spot is your skin, you'll likely experience chronic acne, psoriasis, eczema, or other painful skin conditions. If your vulnerable spot is your gut, you'll likely experience intense bloating, gas, and a slew of digestive discomforts most commonly associated with gluten disorders.

WHAT'S WRONG WITH WHEAT?

I'd be remiss if I didn't talk a bit about what's wrong with wheat today. A lot of people blame "tainted" wheat and the large amounts of it we consume, for the rise in gluten disorders. Is this true?

Americans indeed consume an excess amount of wheat. The U.S. Wheat Associates, an organization that supports the wheat industry and which is partially funded by the USDA, shows wheat consumption is at an all-time high despite the popularity of the gluten-free diet. In fact, human consumption of wheat has increased by 90 million metric tons in the last decade alone.[16] That's a lot of wheat eating if you ask me! Please note that gluten is found in more than just wheat; it's also in barley, rye and spelt. Wheat consumption, however, far surpasses the consumption of other gluten-containing grains by more than a hundred to one,[17] and constitutes 20 percent of all calories consumed.[18]

On top of that, the wheat we eat today is definitely not the same wheat our great grandmothers – and even grandmothers – ate. Dr. William Davis, author of the #1 *New York Times* bestselling book *Wheat Belly*, says that wheat is not genetically modified; rather, it has gone through "countless transformations" due to the crossbreeding and hybridization of wheat.[19] He notes that even small changes in wheat protein structure can "spell the difference between a devastating immune response to wheat protein versus no immune response at all."[20]

In his book, Dr. Davis argues that wheat has been hybridized or crossbred with different strains of wheat and grasses to generate altogether new characteristics and genes. He says farmers covet this high-yielding, semi-dwarf wheat because its short stalks reach maturity quickly, offer a shorter growing season, consume less fertilizer, and result in higher yields.[21] In fact, dwarf and semi-dwarf wheat comprise more than 99 percent of all wheat grown worldwide.[22]

Dr. Davis says that no safety testing has been done to understand the effects of extensive genetic manipulations to wheat and their potential undesirable impacts on humans. He notes that wheat proteins (aka, gluten), in particular, undergo "considerable structural change with hybridization," and in one hybridization experiment, researchers identified fourteen new gluten proteins that were not found in either parent wheat plant. He adds that when you compare modern strains of wheat with wheat of yesteryear, you find modern wheat has a higher number of genes for the gluten proteins associated with celiac disease.[23] In other words, today's wheat contains more gluten than the wheat our ancestors consumed.

It's important to make the distinction that wheat is not genetically modified. Genetic modification means a scientist either inserts or deletes a gene in the wheat's genetic code; rather, our discussion here concerns wheat that has been genetically changed due to hybridization experiments that occurred long before the advent of genetic modification.

WHY THE GLUTEN EPIDEMIC?

It might seem like everyone is or knows someone who has celiac disease or gluten sensitivity these days. What were once rare disorders have somehow gone mainstream. Why?

There are many reasons for the rise in gluten disorders. For starters, awareness of these disorders is at an all-time high among both the medical community and the general population, although arguably we still have a long way to go to fully educate people about the spectrum of gluten disorders. With gluten disorders under an intense public spotlight, a growing number of people are asking their doctors to test them for celiac disease and gluten sensitivities, demanding that their doctors know and do more. Additionally, there is a growing number of direct-to-consumer companies providing screening tests for celiac disease and gluten sensitivity, which people can perform at home. Democratization of testing has more likely than not contributed to the rise in awareness and diagnosis. (Do not diagnose yourself with celiac disease. Discuss the results of any at-home test with your doctor. Only a doctor can diagnose a gluten disorder.)

Researchers are also coming to understand that celiac disease may be afflicting a larger percentage of the population than originally thought, contributing to the "epidemic." While celiac disease is said to affect only one percent of the population, researchers at Children's Hospital Colorado in Denver found this number may be three times higher than originally thought. Researchers tracked 1,339 babies deemed at risk of developing celiac disease and tested each baby annually for the autoimmune disorder over the span of 20 years. In 2015, after 20 years of tracking, researchers reported that more than three percent of the subjects tested positive for celiac disease by the age of 15.[24] As researchers discover that celiac disease affects a larger percentage of the population, doctors will be more likely to screen for it in the future.

In addition to growing awareness, advanced screenings, and greater access to diagnostic tools, many doctors and patients have come to recognize – and accept – that symptoms of gluten disorders go well beyond digestive woes. In fact, there are more than 200 potential symptoms related to celiac disease and gluten sensitivities. More on that in Chapter 2.

However, one disorder that highlights this point is the connection between osteoporosis patients and celiac disease. Osteoporosis is a condition in which the bone becomes less dense and at risk for fractures. More than 53 million people in the U.S. either have or are at high risk for osteoporosis.[25] While many people think they can prevent or combat osteoporosis by consuming more calcium, the truth is that as consumption of calcium increases, so do the rates of osteoporosis.[26] Why is this? The answer is that researchers are finding that osteoporosis may be a complication of untreated celiac disease, among other things. It's not that a patient needs more calcium; it's that they need to split with gluten so they can begin to properly absorb the calcium they're already consuming. Throwing calcium supplements (or worse, a ton of hard-to-digest dairy products – more on this in Part II) at an osteoporosis patient with undiagnosed celiac disease isn't addressing the root cause of their calcium deficiency.

Furthermore, a study published in the *Archives of Internal Medicine* drives home the connection between bone loss and celiac disease. Researchers found that as many as 3-4 percent of osteoporosis patients have untreated celiac disease. Once the researchers put these patients on a gluten-free diet, their bone density dramatically improved.[27] This data shows that doctors should be screening patients for celiac disease at the first sign of bone loss, and is showing us that a slew of symptoms may be caused by undiagnosed celiac disease.

CHAPTER 2
SYMPTOMS OF A GOOD RELATIONSHIP GONE BAD

"You can't connect the dots looking forward; you can only connect them looking backwards. So you have to trust that the dots will somehow connect in your future."

– Steve Jobs

Our bodies contain intricate, interconnected, and inter-dependent systems. What we eat affects every system and organ in our bodies, not just our guts. It's why so many people are not properly diagnosed with a gluten disorder at the first sign of discomfort. For example, if your joints hurt, you visit a rheumatologist. If you suffer from depression, you visit a psychiatrist. If your teeth are broken or decayed, you visit your dentist. If your psoriasis flares up, you visit a dermatologist. No one says, "My joints hurt so I think I'll go to a gastrointestinal doctor to check my small intestine for celiac disease."

We cannot treat symptoms in a bubble, as modern medicine seems determined to do when doctors specialize in treating just one part of the body despite the body being so intricately connected. Instead, I believe we must treat symptoms as a whole and with the recognition that what affects one system or organ in the body starts with the food we eat. Even the great Hippocrates, the Father of Modern Medicine, once said, "All disease begins in the gut." He didn't say *all disease begins in your joints*. He recognized the key role food plays in your overall wellbeing and how what you put in your belly impacts every cell in your body. Maybe instead of seeing your rheumatologist for that nagging joint pain, you should look to your gut for answers.

Unfortunately, it's hard to know if your joint pain is caused by gluten or something else, making diagnosis even more difficult. In fact, there are more than 200 symptoms associated with celiac disease and/or gluten sensitivity, too many to list in this book. That said, common symptoms of celiac disease and/or gluten sensitivity include the following:

Gastrointestinal Symptoms:

- Bloating
- Constipation
- Diarrhea
- Gas
- Foul-smelling stool
- Irritable Bowel Syndrome (IBS)
- Vomiting

Skin Disorders:

- Acne
- Eczema
- Itchy inflamed skin
- Keratosis pilaris (aka chicken skin)
- Psoriasis

Brain Disorders:

- ADHD

- Anxiety
- Autism
- Behavior issues
- Dementia
- Depression
- Headaches
- Irritability
- Migraines

Nutrition-Related Disorders:

- Anemia (iron deficiency)
- Failure to thrive (children)
- Fatigue
- Short stature (children)
- Vitamin deficiencies
- Weakness
- Weight loss

Dental and Mouth Symptoms:

- Canker sores
- Cavities
- Geographic tongue
- Mouth and tongue ulcers
- Tooth enamel defects

Bone, Muscle, and Joint Disorders:

- Arthritis
- Fibromyalgia
- Joint pain and swelling
- Osteopenia (bone loss)
- Osteoporosis
- Recurrent bone fractures

Fertility Issues:

- Infertility
- Low birth weight
- Missed menstrual cycles
- Premature birth
- Recurrent miscarriages

Having one autoimmune disease puts someone at higher risk for other autoimmune diseases. In fact, an estimated 25 percent of patients with one autoimmune disease go on to develop additional autoimmune disorders.[28] A few autoimmune diseases commonly found in patients with gluten disorders include:

- **Dermatitis Herpetiformis (DH):** DH is known as "celiac rash," which is a chronic inflammatory disease of the skin and classified as an autoimmune disease. DH appears in the form of lesions on the skin that burn and itch, and symptoms include symmetrical blisters on the elbows, knees, buttocks, back and/or scalp. The majority of people with DH have the same intestinal damage as seen in those with celiac disease, yet only about 20 percent experience any sort of intestinal symptoms commonly associated with celiac disease.[29]
- **Type 1 Diabetes:** Children with type 1 diabetes are 10-20 times more likely to produce antibodies to wheat and/or have celiac disease, and children with celiac disease are 10 times more likely to develop type 1 diabetes with the risk increasing over time.[30] This means children with type 1 diabetes should be tested for celiac disease, and vice versa, and testing should be performed every few years as both diseases can develop later in life.
- **Inflammatory Bowel Disease (IBD):** People with celiac disease have a nine-fold increased risk of having IBD, a chronic inflammatory disorder that encompasses disorders such as Crohn's and ulcerative colitis.[31]

JENNY LEVINE FINKE

Dr. David Perlmutter dedicated an entire book, *Grain Brain*, a *New York Times* bestseller, to discussing the role of gluten in triggering a slew of brain disorders including dementia, Alzheimer's, epilepsy, headaches, depression, schizophrenia, and ADHD, brushing aside the notion that gluten only affects intestinal health and not neurological wellness.[32] In fact, Dr. Perlmutter says gluten sensitivity "always" affects the brain.[33] If you suffer from any neurological disorder, I highly recommend you read his book to further understand how gluten – and various grains – impact your brain and mental health.

If you have any of the symptoms or disorders listed in this section, please talk to your doctor about getting tested for celiac disease or gluten sensitivity if you haven't already.

CONNECTING THE DOTS

Getting diagnosed with a gluten disorder is a strange thing, in that you begin to connect the dots between gluten and other maladies in your life. While ditching gluten has helped me get my digestive woes under control, it also has contributed to clearing up a slew of deeply personal symptoms, many of which I've experienced my whole life. I used to be embarrassed to talk about my unexplained ailments, but I think doing so can only help others understand that gluten could be the reason behind their *fill-in-the-blank* mystery condition. In the following pages, I share some of the unexplained symptoms I've experienced for years, if not my whole life. Since my split with gluten, these ailments have lessened or gone away. Coincidence? Perhaps. Or maybe gluten is, simply put, behind it all.

Painful Migraines: I used to suffer from painful, intense migraines that usually found me overcome with sickness, sick to my stomach hugging a toilet, and then passed out in a dark room until my symptoms subsided. While I still get minor headaches now and then, I have not had a single migraine since going gluten free. Dot connected. Check.

Geographic Tongue: I used to get these strange, unexplained crop circle-like sores on my tongue known as geographic tongue. These sores were ugly and embarrassing, and they were just worrisome enough that I would ask each of my doctors and dentists over the years if it was anything to be concerned about. Each doctor and dentist told me they didn't know what caused the geographic tongue, and it was nothing of concern. For some reason, in my naiveté, I accepted that explanation. I have since learned that sores on the tongue are a symptom of a nutritional deficiency (a common symptom of unmanaged celiac disease), and geographic tongue is found in 15 percent of patients with celiac disease.[34] I rarely get a geographic tongue flareup anymore, and when I do, it's very minor. Yet another dot connected.

Cold Sores: Like many of my fellow celiac sufferers, I suffered from occasional cold sore outbreaks. I've had cold sores since I was a child and every so often, particularly during times of stress, one would rear its ugly head. Ninety percent of the population has experienced a cold sore or some form of herpes simplex virus in their lifetime.[35] Most people make antibodies to fight future outbreaks, while others, like me, experience recurring cold sores that afflicted me well into adulthood.

It's very painful to talk about having cold sores, as our society has deemed it some sort of taboo sexually transmitted disease. But the truth is, I had a cold sore on my lip long before I ever kissed a boy! I've only had a couple of cold sores since I began the gluten-free diet eight years ago, and one I recall came after I experienced flu-like symptoms.

While I don't have data to support a correlation between cold sores and the gluten-free diet, it can't just be coincidental that this virus dissipated the minute I broke things off with gluten. It's quite possible that my immune system has always been weakened by celiac disease, and viruses love to surface in weakened immune systems. Regardless, this annoying and embarrassing symptom has nearly vanished from my life. Another dot connected.

Keratosis Pilaris: I had these strange, unexplained red and white bumps that would populate the tops of my arm and stay with me day-in and day-out no matter what I did to try to get rid of them. I just lived with the bumps and again, in my naiveté, thought nothing of it. Since saying "so long" to gluten, those pesky bumps have completely disappeared. And while I don't have conclusive research to support a link between celiac disease and keratosis pilaris, I am again connecting the dots and can't help but wonder if ditching gluten had something to do with clearing up these strange bumps.

Low Blood Sugar: I used to be one of those people who had to eat every 2-3 hours or else I would feel weak and shaky. Of course, when I felt weak, I'd always reach for Wheat Thins® or a granola bar. Holy gluten! I now know that I was weak because my body never properly absorbed nutrients from the food I was eating due to unmanaged celiac disease. Again, dots connected. Today I can go hours without eating, and when I'm hungry, I rarely feel shaky or like I'm going to pass out.

TESTING FOR CELIAC DISEASE

Being tested for celiac disease and gluten sensitivity is the only way to know for sure if you suffer from these disorders.

The first step in testing for celiac disease is to request a celiac disease blood test from your doctor. A blood test (a tTG IgA test) is accurate more than 90 percent of the time for those with celiac disease (this is known as "sensitivity" or true positive rate). It can correctly detect a negative result 95 percent of the time (this is known as "specificity" or a true negative rate).[36] This means a blood test is a strong detecting tool for identifying celiac disease in the vast majority of patients. If you receive a positive blood test, for all intents and purposes, you have celiac disease.

Because celiac disease is a life-changing disorder, many doctors recommend that patients who receive a positive celiac test confirm the diagnosis with an endoscopy procedure, where a doctor puts a scope down your throat in order to biopsy your small intestine. (Don't worry, you're under anesthesia and won't feel a thing.) Your doctor is visually looking for damage consistent with celiac disease, which is typically flattened and worn-down microvilli or total villous atrophy. As previously mentioned, the villi are finger-like follicles that surround your small intestine and which are responsible for distributing nutrients from the food you eat to the rest of your body. They play an essential role in proper nutrient absorption. Without fully functioning microvilli, people with celiac disease suffer from nutrient deficiencies and disorders related to malnutrition even if they're eating a "healthy" diet.

You can request a test from your doctor, or take an at-home celiac disease blood test offered by a growing number of companies. The at-home celiac disease test will give you the same reliable results as if your doctor ordered the lab test. You do, however, need to review your results with your doctor as only a doctor can officially "diagnose" you. These at-home tests allow you to do some due diligence first before seeing your doctor. Wouldn't it be great to go to your doctor with confirmed results in hand, ready to discuss next steps? You just may save yourself quite a bit of money, time and headaches involved with multiple doctor visits when you do the test yourself.

If the celiac disease test is negative but you have symptoms that align with the disorder, your doctor may recommend you take a genetic test to see if you carry one of the celiac disease genes. If you do, then your doctor may recommend moving forward with an endoscopy to visually assess and biopsy your small intestine.

My Diagnosis

I was diagnosed with celiac disease after a simple blood test ordered by my primary care doctor. After diagnosis, she suggested I consult with a gastrointestinal doctor to discuss the results and see if further testing would be needed. The GI doctor suggested I have the endoscopy procedure and even flippantly told me that he didn't "think" I had celiac disease because those blood tests are often inaccurate. At the time I believed him because I didn't know any better, but now I realize he was dead wrong.

After my biopsy, my doctor visually confirmed celiac disease and told me he could see damage consistent with celiac disease. A week later, the biopsy results confirmed that I had celiac disease. It was official.

TESTING FOR GLUTEN SENSITIVITY

If you and your doctor have ruled out celiac disease via a blood test, genetic test and biopsy, but symptoms persist, you may want to consider getting tested for gluten sensitivity as the next step. Diagnosing non-celiac gluten sensitivity is challenging, and there isn't a consensus on how to do it. The full-bodied research just isn't here yet; however, don't mistake insufficient research with a non-existent disorder. Gluten sensitivity is a real disorder with real symptoms and real health consequences if left unmanaged or untreated.

Some of the gluten sensitivity tests available as of publication include the Wheat Zoomer test (from Vibrant Wellness) and the Cyrex Array 3 test (from Cyrex Laboratories). These tests evaluate the levels of antibodies to multiple peptides in wheat, not just gliadin, which is the most popular one. Wheat is made up of more than 100 components that can cause a reaction in someone who is sensitive to gluten or wheat.

Many experts say that gluten sensitivity is a precursor to celiac disease. One well-studied biomarker, elevated gliadin-transglutaminase, means you have non-celiac gluten sensitivity and *may* be on the path to developing celiac disease. Elevated gliadin-transglutaminase can be detected up to seven years before someone even develops celiac disease.[37]

ALPHABET SOUP OF TESTS

The testing process can be confusing even for someone knowledgeable about celiac disease. Let's discuss the alphabet soup of tests so you can grow in your knowledge of what each test is looking for.

tTG-IgA and tTG-IgG: There are two types of tTG antibodies that are used to screen for celiac disease: tTG-IgA and tTG-IgG. tTG-IgA antibodies are found in the GI tract and are positive in 95 percent of people with celiac disease. (You must be consuming gluten in order for the test to detect tTG antibodies.) Although rare, about 1-3 percent of the U.S. population is IgA deficient and cannot make IgA antibodies. That's why celiac disease screening also looks for IgG antibodies, which are similar antibodies found throughout the body, not just in the GI tract.

DGP-IgA and DGP-IgG: Celiac disease testing can also include testing for DGP-IgA and DGP-IgG biomarkers. DGP stands for deamidated gliadin peptide and is used to test for celiac disease in people who test negative for tTG antibodies. Gliadin is a protein found in gluten and can be found in the body *before* tTG antibodies are present. DGP tests may someday aid in the early detection of celiac disease, especially in children.[38]

Immunoglobulin G (IgG): Food sensitivity tests are looking for immunoglobulin G (IgG) antibodies. IgG antibodies bind to food and account for 75 percent of the antibodies circulating in your blood. Antibodies are an important part of your body's response to toxins because they recognize and bind to particular antigens, such as bacteria or viruses, and then help to destroy those toxins. It's important to note that an IgG test is a test for food sensitivity only, not food allergy. Unfortunately, the terms "food sensitivity" and "food allergy" are mistakenly used interchangeably, adding to the confusion. See Chapter 13 for more information on testing for food sensitivities.

Immunoglobulin E (IgE): IgE antibodies are produced by your immune system and show your immune system's overreaction to a specific allergen. It is the test used for detecting a true allergy to wheat (or other allergen). IgE antibodies travel to your cells and release chemicals that cause an allergic reaction.

A POTENTIAL SNAG IN THE PLAN

In order to be tested for celiac disease or gluten sensitivity, you must be consistently eating gluten. This is tricky because a lot of people implement the gluten-free diet first to see if they feel better without ruling out celiac disease via a simple blood test. One of my blog readers emailed to tell me her doctor had told her to *try the gluten-free diet* to see if she felt better without doing any tests first. She stopped eating gluten and started to feel a lot better. She later tried to reintroduce gluten in order to get tested for celiac disease, and she told me she couldn't do it because eating gluten was a painful proposition. "I will never eat gluten again," she lamented. If only her doctor had given her a simple celiac disease blood test *before* advising her to ditch gluten, she would have known if she had celiac disease or gluten sensitivity. Now she may never know.

If you've already broken up with gluten before ruling out celiac disease, you have several options to find out whether you have celiac disease or gluten sensitivity.

The first thing you can do is get tested for celiac disease even if you're following a gluten-free diet. While you must be eating gluten in order for the test to be accurate, six out of ten people who are already following a gluten-free diet and who take a celiac disease test will still see elevated antibodies to the peptides in gluten.[39] This is likely due, unfortunately, to the fact that most people on a gluten-free diet are still eating trace amounts of gluten on a continuous basis. Some people test positive despite their best efforts to eat gluten free, due to the high burden of limiting even the tiniest exposure to gluten.

If the celiac disease test is negative, and you still have symptoms concurrent with the disorder, consider taking a genetic test to see if you carry one of the two celiac disease genes – HLA DQ2 or DQ8. About 30 percent of the population carries one of the genes associated with celiac disease, but only three to five percent of those who carry one or both of the genes will go on to develop celiac disease.[40] If you don't have the HLA DQ2 or DQ8 genes, then you don't have celiac disease. However, if you have one of the two celiac disease genes, you may want to move on to the next level of testing, which requires you to take what is aptly called the "Gluten Challenge."

THE GLUTEN CHALLENGE

The Gluten Challenge is where you reintroduce gluten into your diet consistently for a period of time in order to take – and get an accurate result for – a celiac disease test. Experts generally recommend that you eat three to ten grams of gluten per day for six to eight weeks or the equivalent of two to four slices of bread each day (a slice of bread is about two grams),[41] although some experts say you need to be eating gluten for closer to 12 weeks. The bottom line is you need to be eating a meaningful amount of gluten consistently for a prolonged period of time in order for a celiac disease test to be accurate.

The process of adding gluten back into your diet can be a painful one, especially if you are symptomatic to gluten. That said, I understand why someone would want to put themselves through the Gluten Challenge.

For starters, many people want to know *for sure* if they have celiac disease vs. gluten sensitivity. When they are certain they have celiac disease, they may feel like they will be taken more seriously by friends, families, waiters, and even the medical community. Unfortunately, gluten sensitivity, although a very real and serious disorder, isn't as widely accepted in today's society, and unfortunately it's questioned, dismissed, and made fun of by many, including late night comics.

Furthermore, diagnosed celiac patients are more likely to strictly adhere to the gluten-free diet, which will serve them well over the long-term. People diagnosed with non-celiac gluten sensitivity may be more lackadaisical in the management of their diet and perhaps not as concerned about cross-contamination. I can't tell you how many of my gluten-sensitive friends have said to me, "While I eat gluten free and generally avoid gluten, I don't have anything as serious as celiac disease, so I don't have to be as cautious when I eat out."

On top of that, being tested for celiac disease helps research-ers paint a more accurate picture of the actual number of people afflicted. If someone goes gluten free before first ruling out celiac disease, we may never know the true prevalence of the disorder.

Interestingly enough, in 2016 researchers at Rutgers University found the rates of celiac diagnosis stagnant for the first time since 2009.[42] This number is likely skewed, however, due to people self-diagnosing their conditions and choosing to follow a gluten-free diet without *first* ruling out celiac disease. When someone isn't first tested for celiac disease, it becomes impossible to determine the true prevalence of the disorder; researchers may falsely conclude that the number of people with celiac disease is decreasing.

Should researchers find the number of cases of celiac disease on the rise, and the "true" number of people afflicted with the disorder comes to full light, interest from researchers, doctors, and pharmaceutical companies will increase. While more research and money is needed to understand and treat celiac disease and gluten sensitivities, this will only happen if the disorders afflict a larger percentage of the population and thereby make it finan-cially worthwhile for researchers to study.

Lastly, celiac disease patients may be eligible for future treat-ments or benefits, but they must have an official diagnosis to qualify. (Perhaps one day there will be treatment options – a medication or vaccine, both of which researchers are working toward – beyond the gluten-free diet for those of us with celiac disease.) This also means that should additional insurance benefits become available for those with diagnosed celiac disease, as they are in some countries outside the U.S., those on a gluten-free diet without a celiac disease diagnosis wouldn't be able to take advantage of those benefits without an official diagnosis. Italy, for example, offers a stipend to pay for gluten-free food for people with celiac disease in order to offset the added costs associated with the lifestyle.

Don't Want to Take the Challenge?

The reality is that whether you have celiac disease or gluten sensitivity, the current treatment is exactly the same. At the end of the Gluten Challenge, all you have to show for it is a confirmed diagnosis (or not) and a (re)damaged intestine that may take many months, even years, to heal and put back into remission. You might be doing more harm than good when you go back on gluten *just* to be tested.

Ultimately, deciding whether or not to take the Gluten Challenge is a personal decision. There is no right or wrong answer. However, before reintroducing gluten into your diet, consider being genetically tested for celiac disease first, as well as undergoing a celiac disease blood test to see if gluten antibodies are detectable. Regardless of your decision, I hope you find the answers you're looking for and peace with your decision and the outcome.

IT TAKES GUTS: THE MARATHON MOTHER GIVES UP GLUTEN

Beatie Deutsch is a national marathon champion based in Israel. In 2016, Deutsch placed sixth in her first marathon ever, the Tel Aviv Marathon, having taken up running only four months prior. She later ran the 2017 Tel Aviv Marathon while seven months pregnant and the Jerusalem Marathon in March 2018. However, one month before the Jerusalem marathon run, Deutsch became very weak and fatigued. She didn't know why.

"I had been training for several months, running six times a week and giving it my all; but instead of feeling like things were progressing, I felt weaker," she recalls. "I remember coming back after my first 20-miler completely and totally depleted, as if I was retracting from my goal. I blamed the Jerusalem course for being such a killer course."

The fatigue continued to plague the marathon mother, and that's when she says she knew something was "off." After checking in with her doctor and running a few blood tests, Deutsch found out she was severely anemic.

"I remember feeling down. My training until that point had all been compromised. It was now five weeks before the marathon. My hemoglobin was around seven (extremely low), and it felt like all my goals were headed down the drain."

Deutsch, 28 years old at the time, suspected celiac disease might be the root cause of her anemia; after all, her four siblings have it. And while she tested negative for celiac disease in the past, she knew celiac disease can *turn on* at any time. Within a week of finding out she was anemic, Deutsch also tested positive for celiac disease.

Despite this setback, Deutsch admits she chose to "focus on the positive," and continually reminded herself how grateful she was to have figured out the issue so quickly. While she could have quit or felt sorry for herself, she decided to stay optimistic. She still had five weeks to get her act together before the Jerusalem Marathon – no time for a pity party!

"There will always be setbacks on our journeys, and the most important thing is how we handle those challenges and whether we let them knock us down or not," she says. She adds that she chose to accept this as part of God's plan for her; and if things didn't work out at the Jerusalem Marathon as she hoped, there would be other opportunities to try again and win in a different year.

Deutsch did everything she could to rebound quickly and turn her health around. She had an iron infusion and immediately implemented the gluten-free diet.

"I honestly really wanted to just stuff my face with all the gluten I could for one more day, but I knew that would only harm me so I restrained myself," she admits. She says she was determined to get back to running and had no time to waste.

"When I showed up at the start line [at the Jerusalem Marathon], I had no idea whether I'd be able to achieve my goal, but I knew I would give it my all. I held on to my mantra to stay positive because at the end of the day, when things don't work out, the only thing that can really help us is to keep smiling and realize it's all part of God's plan. Whether you're running through life or just taking a stroll, everything is always better when you're smiling," she says.

Deutsch went on to beat the odds, coming in first place in the Jerusalem Marathon with a time of 3:09 and setting a course record for all female runners. The next year she won first place at the Israeli National Championships Marathon in Tiberias with a time of 2:42, the fifth best time for all-time female Israeli runners. She now has her sights set on the 2021 Summer Olympics.

Deutsch concurs that eating gluten free has made it easier to eat healthy and stay disciplined while she's training because there aren't nearly as many gluten-free treats and options available, and today she sees the elimination of gluten as a "necessary component" to getting healthy and in tip-top shape.

CHAPTER 3
GLUTEN, I'M ON TO YOU

"The most important thing to remember about food labels
is that you should avoid foods that have labels."

– Dr. Joel Fuhrman

The biggest question most people have after breaking up with gluten is what in the world are they going to eat? They've been eating certain foods for so long, and now, at the flip of a switch, everything must change. (I do mean everything!)

You must learn to sniff out gluten wherever you go. Gluten is found in wheat, rye, barley, spelt, and some oats (more on oats in a bit). But there are some not-so-obvious hiding places where your ex likes to lurk.

Of course, you should avoid the obvious gluten hangouts, like bread, pasta, pizza, donuts, pastries, breadcrumbs, and croutons. These foods look doughy and gluten-y. But what you may not realize is that so many foods don't "look" like gluten yet contain plenty of the damaging protein inside. My ex was going to be harder to shake than I first realized.

Gluten comes in many shapes and forms. Beyond wheat, rye and barley, the following are just some of the many names gluten goes by:

- Abyssinian Hard (wheat)
- Bulgur (whole wheat grain)
- Dextrin (may be derived from wheat, corn or tapioca – check labels)
- Durum (type of hard wheat)
- Einkorn (wheat)
- Farina (milled wheat)
- Fu (wheat gluten)
- Groats (cereal kernels or "berries" made from wheat, barley, rye or oat)
- Hydrolyzed vegetable protein (may contain wheat, barley or soy)
- Kamut (ancient wheat)
- Maida (finely milled wheat flour from India)
- Malt (flavoring and vinegar both typically contain barley)
- Secale (rye)
- Seitan (tofu-like meat substitute made from vital wheat gluten)
- Semolina (purified durum wheat)
- Spelt (form of wheat)
- Triticale or Triticum (all forms of wheat hybrids)
- Wild Emmer (wheat hybrid)

These are some of the *not-so-obvious* products where gluten is *typically* found:

- BBQ sauces
- Beer (and brewer's yeast)
- Bouillon cubes
- Broths
- Caramel color (barley malt)
- Couscous

- Gravies
- Gummy bears and gummy candies
- Imitation crab and bacon
- Licorice
- Onion soup mix
- Orzo
- Pearled couscous
- Play-Doh™ (while you don't eat it, you touch it and it gets under your nails and *could* be transferred to your food.)
- Rice Krispies™ (contains barley malt)
- Salad dressings
- Sourdough bread (more on this later)
- Soy sauce or shoyu
- Tabbouleh (made from bulger)
- Worcestershire sauce (unless labeled GF or gluten free)

CONFUSING LABELS

I bet you didn't know that being diagnosed with a gluten disorder means you have to become a master label reader. You have to know so much information about strange ingredients, like maltodextrin and yeast extract, and understand, with certainty, whether these ingredients are gluten free. Let's take some time discussing labels so you can up your label-reading game and avoid your ex like the plague!

GLUTEN LABELING

Most mainstream and specialty food manufacturers are good about labeling their products as "gluten free." Personally, I look for the gluten-free label whenever I shop. Unfortunately, however, label reading is not foolproof and manufacturers – and consumers – make mistakes.

While most products labeled "gluten free" abide by the FDA's guidelines for gluten-free labeling (more on that in a bit), there may be times when you want to try a product that is not labeled "gluten free." This is when you have to be extra vigilant and scrutinize the ingredient labels and manufacturer disclosures. Even a product that does not contain any gluten or questionable ingredients might still contain gluten because the product, or the raw ingredients used to make the product, somehow came in contact with gluten along the way. It's rare, but possible.

I like to consider myself a master gluten-sniffer-outer, but even I've been fooled. After carefully reviewing the ingredients of a package of organic chocolate pudding, and deeming it "safe," it still made me sick. How could this be? While the product wasn't labeled "gluten free," I didn't see any questionable ingredients. I decided to test the pudding for gluten using a portable gluten-detecting device, which I will tell you more about in Chapter 5. As suspected by my body's visceral reaction to the pudding, the test came back positive for gluten.

I share this story to show you why I think it's always best to opt for products labeled "gluten free." When a product bears the gluten-free label, in theory it meets FDA guidelines, which require gluten-free labeled products to contain less than 20 parts per million (ppm) of gluten. Twenty ppm is a minute amount (0.002 percent). The FDA says this trace amount is safe for someone with celiac disease to consume without causing intestinal damage. It's important to note, however, that the FDA set this legal limit based on the technology available in 2013 and based on information gleaned from a study about how much gluten a person with celiac disease could tolerate without getting sick. Labeling a product as "gluten free" is 100 percent voluntary and self-regulated. If a company chooses to make a gluten-free claim on its label, it must abide by the FDA's guidelines. If consumers become sick from a product labeled "gluten free," they should report it to the FDA for investigation.

As mentioned, some products are mistakenly labeled "gluten free." I have two recent examples of this happening, both with supplements (read those supplement labels carefully, friends!). One supplement had a label that said "No gluten." I assumed the product would be safe for me to consume. However, upon further inspection, I noticed it contained oat grass. I inquired of the company, which provided me with its gluten test results: 40 ppm of gluten, double the legal limit! The company acknowledged its error and has since corrected it.

A woman in my gluten-free diet support group on Facebook showed a picture of a digestive enzyme bottle that clearly says "No gluten" on the label. Upon further investigation, I noticed the allergen disclosure statement says, "Contains wheat ingredients." What?!? I told her to contact the company for clarification, as well as report the product to an FDA Consumer Complaint Coordinator. Both of these examples are cautionary tales that gluten will try to sneak back into your life when you least expect it.

An added layer of confidence comes only with products labeled "certified gluten free." These certifying standards are set by third-party, non-regulatory agencies. The Gluten-Free Certification Organization (GFCO) is the largest certifying agency in the U.S. Manufacturers pay the GFCO, and other certifying organizations, to periodically audit their ingredients and practices, which allows use of the organization's trademarked logo on their packaging. Each independent agency has its own set of certifying standards. The GFCO, for example, only certifies products that test at 10 ppm or less of gluten, which is a lower threshold than the 20 ppm required by the FDA. Becoming certified gluten free is also voluntary for manufacturers, and I can personally speak to having more confidence in a product that has been third-party certified, particularly in today's wild-west labeling practices.

ALLERGEN LABELING

Eight allergens account for nearly 90 percent of all food allergies in the United States. These allergens include milk, eggs, fish, shellfish, tree nuts, peanuts, wheat, and soy. In the U.S., these allergens must be declared on the packaging of processed food as set forth by the Food Allergen Labeling and Consumer Protection Act of 2004.

While the FDA classifies wheat as a top allergen, gluten is not technically an "allergen." In fact, as you have learned, gluten is found in more than just wheat; it's also in barley, rye, spelt, and sometimes oats. Unfortunately, the FDA does not require manufacturers to list all gluten-containing ingredients on their allergen disclosure statements, so you should not rely solely on allergen disclosure statements to determine if a product is free from gluten. I learned this the hard way early on in my gluten-free journey when I thought I could eat a fun-size 100 Grand Bar®. The allergen disclosure label read, "Contains milk and soy ingredients. May contain peanut and egg ingredients." I didn't see wheat listed, so I thought I was in the clear to indulge in this treat. Wrong! I failed to read the ingredient label; if I had, I would have clearly seen that the candy bar contained barley malt. This incident reminded me to always carefully read both the ingredient list and the allergen statements before enjoying any packaged food.

CONFUSING DISCLOSURE STATEMENTS

Sometimes packaged goods will have a disclosure statement that says, "May Contain Wheat." This statement generally has one of four meanings:

1. It may mean the product has no "gluten" ingredients but the final product has not been independently verified by the manufacturer nor certified by a third-party organization.
2. It may mean the raw ingredients used to make the packaged food item have not been independently verified as gluten free.
3. It may mean the product is produced on shared equipment that has touched gluten so there may have been potential cross-contact with gluten during the manufacturing process.

4. It may mean the product is produced in the same facility as products that contain wheat, even if in a separate room and on separate equipment.

Unfortunately, there are all sorts of confusing labels in the industry. These statements are voluntarily made by the manufacturer and not required by law. The manufacturer, however, is telling us something to the effect that it doesn't know if the product contains gluten, but it's possible. In their effort to be more transparent, they are confusing the heck out of us!

You'll also see other voluntary label disclosures such as, "Processed on equipment shared with wheat," or "Contains no gluten ingredients."

Food products that are processed on equipment shared with wheat are off-limits in my book. While manufacturing lines are usually cleaned between the manufacturing of each product, the possibility of food coming in contact with bits of wheat is possible and even probable.

A disclosure of "Contains no gluten ingredients" should also have you looking for additional clues to help you decide whether the product is safe for you to eat. Before consuming the product, consider contacting the manufacturer to find out why it put that statement on its packaging. Is it because wheat is being used for other products manufactured in its facility, or is it because it has not verified how the sourced ingredients were handled before it received them?

Finally, one other confusing statement manufacturers typically include, even on products labeled "gluten free" or "certified gluten free," is: "Manufactured in the same facility as wheat." The "same facility" could mean that wheat is being handled in a separate room down the hall, or on a manufacturing line next to the one producing the gluten-free item. When I eat at a restaurant or friend's house and when I ate in my kitchen before it became a dedicated gluten-free kitchen, my food would have been considered "manufactured" in the same facility as foods that contain gluten. Many times, after careful inspection of the label and research, I will feel comfortable eating products manufactured in the same facility as wheat as long as it's not produced on the same equipment. That said, I do so on a case-by-case basis and only after I put much thought and due diligence into that decision. If the product is labeled "gluten free" or certified gluten free, and unless you are anaphylaxis allergic to wheat, it's more likely than not okay for you to eat. If the product causes you to become sick, report it immediately to the FDA.

CONFUSING INGREDIENTS

While label reading can be extremely difficult at the start of your gluten-free journey, it does become easier with time. Following are some ingredients on labels that you will want to take special note of as you attempt to decode gluten *free* from gluten *full*:

Maltodextrin: Maltodextrin is a food additive found in many processed foods. The word itself is confusing because it contains the word "malt," which is typically associated with barley. Maltodextrin is safe to consume on a gluten-free diet, even if derived from wheat,[43] because maltodextrin is highly processed to the point that the gluten is removed. On top of that, the vast majority of maltodextrin used in processed foods comes from corn or tapioca, not from wheat.

Vinegar: Another ingredient that stumps gluten-free eaters is vinegar. Regular *distilled* vinegar is gluten free. Wine and grape vinegar (distilled from grapes), and apple cider vinegar (distilled from apples) are also gluten free. Fully distilled "pure" vinegar is 100 percent gluten free even if it's derived from wheat, barley or rye.[44] However, if you're using *non-distilled* vinegar, you must read the label carefully. If the non-distilled vinegar is made from wheat, barley, or rye as its starting material, then the vinegar is not free from gluten. Flavored vinegars, particularly malt vinegars, are typically derived from barley and may contain gluten.

Modified Food Starch: Most modified food starch is made from corn or potato; however, it also can come from wheat. Due to required FDA food labeling in the U.S., if modified food starch comes from wheat, the word "wheat" must be listed somewhere on the ingredient label or allergen disclosure statement. If you don't see the statement, the modified food starch is most likely free from gluten, although to be on the safe side you should contact the manufacturer to confirm the source of the starch.

Alcohol: Ask ten people whether alcohol is gluten free, and you will receive ten different answers. Even I'm confused by it. Many people have different comfort levels as to what they will – and won't – drink. Let's take a moment to *distill* the facts.

Distilled vs. Fermented:

First, it's important to note that all distilled liquor is *technically* gluten free even if distilled from a gluten-containing grain, as the distillation process removes the gluten protein from the final product.[45] This means distilled spirits, such as vodka, gin, whisky, brandy, rum and tequila, are deemed gluten free.

However, it's another story if a beverage is fermented, which includes wine, beer, wine coolers, hard cider and hard lemonade. If the starting ingredient contains gluten, like wheat, barley or rye, then the fermented beverage is not free from gluten. However, if the starting material is corn, grapes or other fruit, then such beverages are considered gluten free.

Labeling Laws:

There are very specific regulations on how an alcoholic beverage can be labeled.

The Alcohol and Tobacco Tax and Trade Bureau (TTB), the government agency that regulates liquor, says that alcoholic beverages made from non-gluten containing ingredients, such as wines fermented from grapes or other fruit, and distilled spirits distilled from potato or corn, can make "gluten-free" claims on their labels.

However, the FDA says any product distilled from a gluten ingredient, such as wheat, barley and rye, even if the gluten is removed (such is the case with "gluten-removed beers"), cannot be labeled "gluten free." Gluten removed means a beverage was distilled from a gluten-containing grain such as wheat, but that the wheat was processed, treated, or crafted to remove the gluten protein from the final product. Unfortunately, there is no way to confirm that the final product is free from gluten, so experts generally advise people with celiac and gluten sensitivities to steer clear of gluten-removed beers and beverages.

Flavors:

Sometimes manufacturers add flavoring after the distillation process, as in the case of flavored liqueurs. You'll not only want to know the grain source for the liqueur, but also if any of the added flavoring(s) contain gluten. I personally err on the side of caution and only drink unflavored alcohol distilled from gluten-free grains.

Everyone can make their own decision on whether or not they feel comfortable drinking distilled alcoholic beverages that are made from wheat, barley or rye, and whether they feel comfortable drinking a fermented beverage labeled "gluten-removed."

To help you make that decision, I've compiled a list of spirits derived from gluten-y ingredients vs. gluten-free ingredients:

Spirits distilled from gluten-containing grains:

- Bourbon may be distilled from corn, rye, malted barley or wheat.
- Gin is typically distilled from wheat, rye or barley, however, some gin is distilled from corn or potato.
- Scotch is distilled from malted barley, maize (corn) or wheat.
- Vodka is typically distilled from wheat or rye, however, some vodka is distilled from corn, sorghum or potato.
- Whiskey is distilled from barley, corn, rye or wheat.

Spirits that are naturally gluten free:

- Brandy is typically distilled from grapes.

- Cognac is typically distilled from white wine (grapes).
- Rum is distilled from sugar cane.
- Tequila is distilled from the agave plant.

Brown Rice Syrup: Brown rice syrup goes by the names "rice syrup" or "rice malt" and is typically made by soaking cooked rice starch with sprouted barley enzymes – yikes! If a product contains brown rice syrup and is labeled "gluten free," then you know that barley enzymes were not used. However, if the product contains brown rice syrup and is not labeled "gluten free," you should definitely avoid it.

Wheatgrass: Wheatgrass is technically gluten free despite its name, but deciding whether you should eat it while on a gluten-free diet isn't an easy call. Wheatgrass juice is extracted from the freshly sprouted first leaves of the wheat plant before the wheat seed begins to form. The seed, which forms at about day 17 of a wheat sprout's life, is where the protein (gluten) resides. This means if you're eating the grass (without the seed), then you're consuming the gluten-free part of the plant. You are, however, trusting that the farmer growing the wheatgrass has a purely wheatgrass farm and that he or she has been mindful of the harvesting and production process to ensure no seeds infiltrate the final product. You have no way of telling if the farmer took such care during the processing of commercially produced wheatgrass, and this is why I personally avoid wheatgrass unless it's found in a product that has been certified gluten free. Of course, if you have a wheat allergy, avoid wheatgrass whether or not the seed is present.

Barley Grass: Barley grass is also gluten free, but the seed is not. See "Wheatgrass."

Gelatin: Gelatin sounds a lot like gluten; however, gelatin is gluten free as it's the collagen of animal bones, such as cows, pigs, fish, and is used as a gelling agent in food products. It's most notably found in Jell-O™, marshmallows, and gummies (including gummy vitamins). While vegans avoid gelatin because it's derived from animal parts, gelatin itself is gluten free.

Natural Flavors: Natural flavors is a catch-all ingredient found in many processed foods. Most natural flavors are gluten free unless noted on the ingredient label; however, look for products labeled "gluten free" to be on the safe side.

MSG: Monosodium glutamate, commonly known as MSG, is a flavor-enhancing food additive that gives food a savory, desirable taste known as "umami" in Japanese. While various starches are used in making MSG, it's rarely sourced from wheat. To be safe, look for products labeled "gluten free" when MSG is present. Keep in mind, however, that the MSG additive has been linked to various forms of toxicity, including "gastric distension," so it might be wise to avoid it altogether.[46]

Oats: Oats are naturally gluten free; however, they are often grown in fields in rotation with wheat crops. This means the same fields are used in harvesting the crops, and the same processing and storage equipment is used for both grains.

You can purchase safe, gluten-free oats from reputable brands. Some brands use "purity protocol oats," which are oats grown on dedicated gluten-free fields and processed using dedicated gluten-free equipment. Other brands produce what is called "commodity" oats, which means the manufacturer optically or mechanically sorts and scrubs their oats to remove any traces of wheat so only the oat grain is left.

Many people in the celiac community disagree over whether commodity oats are safe. I personally take my lead from the North American Society for the Study of Celiac Disease (NASSCD), the organization that represents the continent's leading celiac disease researchers. NASSCD says that regardless of whether the oats are purity or commodity oats, there must be "rigorous" and "precise" validation testing and transparent results available to the public for scrutiny; such results should consistently guarantee the oats contain less than 20 ppm of gluten.[47] In other words, if a manufacturer is able to instill consumer confidence in the oats due to valid and strict manufacturing and testing measures, commodity oats are fine to consume.

Sourdough: Well-meaning friends might tell you that you can still eat sourdough wheat bread because fermentation breaks down the gluten to the extent that it is no longer detectable. While it is true that fermentation breaks down the gluten protein, making sourdough more easily digestible by humans, you would be hard-pressed to find sourdough prepared in a safe way even by the most skilled sourdough bakers. Sourdough bread, for all intents and purposes, contains gluten and is cross-contaminated with gluten at some point during processing. Only sourdough bread made from gluten-free grains (and using a gluten-free starter) is safe to consume on a gluten-free diet.

Yeast: Most people associate yeast with bread and don't realize it's gluten free and safe to eat. In fact, you need yeast (or a gluten-free sourdough starter) to make gluten-free bread or pizza dough.

Yeast Extract: While yeast is gluten free, yeast extract may not be. Yeast extract and autolyzed yeast extract are often made from spent brewer's yeast. Spent brewer's yeast is a byproduct of the brewing process and most likely contains wheat or other gluten-containing grains. Unless you know the source of yeast extract or a product is labeled "gluten free," avoid it.

It Takes Guts: Dana Vollmer Puts Her Carb-Loading Days in the Past

Dana Vollmer is a four-time Olympic gold medalist and world-record setting swimming champion. This elite athlete says eliminating gluten, along with eggs, helped her reach new heights in her swimming career. In fact, she says it was her breakup with gluten that propelled her elite athletic performance at the 2012 Summer Olympics where she set the 100-meter butterfly world record and walked away with three gold medals.

"I had stomach aches from before I can even remember. A lot of them were at swim meets and it hurt to just put on my swimsuit. My parents would sit in the car with me at competitions and massage my stomach. I even went to the emergency room twice, thinking my appendix had burst. I'm a tough athlete and have a high pain tolerance. Doctors would just diagnose me with constipation and gas, but I knew it was something more."

Vollmer's chronic stomach aches persisted, and it finally prompted her to reach out to a nutritionist to get answers her doctor could not provide. Her nutritionist tested her for celiac disease, food allergies, and food sensitivities. The tests revealed that she had sensitivities to gluten and eggs. Now she finally understood why she was in so much pain at competitions.

"I had been carb-loading before the swim meets thinking it was good for me," she says. Ironically, all that carb-loading (aka gluten-loading) was the exact thing causing her so much pain!

Since dumping gluten, she says she feels amazing. If gluten accidentally slips into her diet, she says her body instantly swells up and she experiences bad headaches and constipation for several days. These natural consequences have helped her realize that there's no room for gluten in her life as a competitive swimmer and busy mother of two young children.

"I've come to realize that while I don't have celiac disease, gluten has still caused a lot of pain in my life. I feel so much better without it and I feel like I shouldn't have to defend that it's *just* a food sensitivity. I tell people new to breaking up with gluten to give it time and be gentle with themselves. It's hard to flip a switch and say I'm completely over you. It's a process of figuring out what we like and figuring out a new routine. It gets easier with time."

CHAPTER 4
CONSCIOUSLY UNCOUPLING

"Before you heal someone, ask him if he's willing to give up the things that make him sick."

– Hippocrates

Now that you have a better understanding of where gluten lurks, it's time to focus on getting it out of your house – and life – for good.

Freeing your body of gluten is more complicated if you share your kitchen with gluten eaters, as you can't force others to split with gluten too. This is why it's essential to create space and boundaries. Others can continue to "see" gluten; they just need to respect that you and gluten have called it quits.

GETTING STARTED

Dedicate a morning or afternoon to rummaging through your pantry and fridge. Sort everything into three piles: (1) Gluten (2) Gluten Free and (3) Not Sure. Sorting your food into piles can be a humbling experience, and it might make you sad or regretful. These are normal emotions. It can feel like you're boxing up your ex's belongings. I remember feeling a strong sense of loss at that time. I also started to blame myself as if I had brought on my celiac disease myself by all the gluten, sugary, and processed foods I ate. Don't be hard on yourself. You didn't see it coming. That is the past. When you know better, you can do better. This is a new beginning in your life.

After you sort your piles and determine what is and isn't gluten free, you'll want to designate space in your refrigerator and pantry for your gluten-free items. Be sure to first thoroughly wipe down the shelves. I reserve the two top shelves in my pantry for my foodstuffs to keep my food out of easy reach from the gluten eaters in my house; and, should something spill, like cereal, I don't want it to leak onto or mix with my precious gluten-free foods. You'll also want to label your food items and shelves, and explain your setup to the gluten eaters in your home.

Here are a few other tips to setting up your kitchen in a way that supports your new life sans gluten:

- Label all gluten-free items as "gluten free," particularly items you don't want gluten-y hands getting into. You can print labels and stick them on top of your items, or use a good old Sharpie to clearly mark everything. I also have chip clips that say "Gluten Free" to help my family know not to stick their gluten-y hands into my bags of chips or popcorn.
- Wipe down the inside of all your kitchen drawers and cabinets. There are likely gluten crumbs lingering in your silverware drawer.
- Purchase your own condiments – butter, mayo, peanut butter, jelly, etc. Think about how your son might dip his knife in the butter tub, then spread the butter on top of toast, and then dip the knife back into the butter tub to grab more. You don't want gluten-y crumbs contaminating your gluten-free butter.
- Purchase a new toaster, a few new pots and pans, a couple of new spatulas, and a new strainer/colander; such items will be used only for gluten-free cooking. The kitchen

items you have been using will have gluten-y residue and should be tossed or reserved for those that still mingle with gluten. To avoid confusion, I bought these items in red, offering a visual clue to those in my house that the red item is the gluten-free toaster and colander. I also stored my new color-coded items on my dedicated pantry shelves so others wouldn't confuse them with the gluten-y kitchen tools. Of course, if your kitchen ever becomes a dedicated gluten-free kitchen one day, you'll simply clean everything well, replace items that need to be fresh, and then everything will be fine for use by everyone. I shared my kitchen with the gluten eaters in my family for the first three years post-breakup; however, today my kitchen is dedicated gluten free. No gluten is prepared or eaten on my dishes anymore. Ironically, this was a decision my husband made (not me) after he saw me struggle to feel safe eating in my own home. It was the best decision ever but one that we came to, as a family, over time.

- Have a separate sponge for cleaning your gluten-free pots and pans. I used to have a pink sponge (couldn't find a red one) just for cleaning gluten-free items, and I had a blue sponge for washing gluten-y pots and pans. Again, colors offer visual clues to your family on what items they can use for gluten vs. gluten-free items. Consider having color-coded dish towels too.

COOKING

While I *now* know that eating gluten free is no big deal, it was an all-consuming and overwhelming task when I was first figuring it all out. I truly felt paralyzed in the kitchen.

My first night post-diagnosis was the worst. I had planned on making spaghetti with meat sauce; but I had only gluten-y spaghetti in the house, and I didn't know if the jarred spaghetti sauce I had been using all these years was gluten free. That night I made one meal for my family, then a separate meal – a scrambled egg and apple – for myself. It was a humbling experience. I wish I had been kinder to myself back then; I wish I had known that I was just at the start line of a very long marathon that would continue for the rest of my life. The first hours, days, and weeks are the hardest. I kept reminding myself, this too shall pass.

Remember, even though you've split with gluten, there are still so many foods you *can* eat. The safest, and arguably best, foods for you to eat are foods that are naturally gluten free. When you eat foods that don't come in a package or bear an ingredient label, you won't have to worry about gluten. Below are some of the naturally gluten-free foods you can enjoy without worry:

- **Fresh Vegetables and Fruits:** You can eat any fruit or vegetable on the planet. Enjoy apples, bananas, kale, avocados, celery sticks, and the full rainbow of fresh produce.
- **Fresh Meats:** Fresh meat is gluten free. Enjoy baked chicken thighs, grilled steak, or roasted pork chops. If a meat item is packaged or prepared, like hot dogs or deli meats, be sure to check the labels for hidden gluten. Avoid sliced meats from the deli counter and opt for packaged meats instead to avoid the potential for cross contamination.
- **Fresh Fish:** You can safely enjoy fresh fish like salmon, halibut or tilapia, and fresh shellfish like shrimp and crab. Top fish with a little oil, salt and pepper, and fresh seasonings for delicious flavor and no worry of gluten. Canned salmon and tuna are free from gluten, although read labels to verify.
- **Fresh Dairy:** Most fresh cheeses are free from gluten. Just beware of blue cheese; it is typically gluten free although some experts say the mold cultures for this type of cheese are grown on wheat or rye bread. You'll also want to be conscientious when eating pre-shredded cheese and cheese spreads. Check labels for ingredients and allergen disclosures. (You can always buy a block of cheese and shred it yourself to be on the safe side.) Butter and milk are

also naturally gluten free, although, as we'll talk about in Chapter 13, many people who eat gluten cannot tolerate dairy products.

- **Nuts and Seeds:** Nuts and seeds are perfect for snacking and are naturally gluten free. If packaged, read the ingredients and manufacturer processing disclosures carefully. Never buy these items from the bulk bins as the risk of cross-contact with gluten is too high.
- **Gluten-Free Grains:** Rice, corn, buckwheat, millet, and quinoa (technically a seed) are all gluten-free grains. Oats are naturally gluten free but they are cross-contaminated with wheat during the harvesting and manufacturing processes. If you want to enjoy oats, they need to come in packaging labeled "gluten free." Avoid getting grains from the bulk bins as well.

The following grains and starches are naturally gluten free:

Amaranth	Potato
Arrowroot	Quinoa
Buckwheat	Rice
Cassava	Sorghum
Corn, including hominy, cornmeal, grits and polenta	Soy
Flax	Tapioca
Millet	Teff

- **Eggs:** Eggs are naturally gluten free and are also the most bioavailable food on the planet. Bioavailability means your body knows how to use all the nutrients found inside the food.
- **Potatoes:** Potatoes are naturally gluten free. French fries are also gluten free (thank goodness!). If fries prepared by a restaurant are deep fried in the same cooking oil as

items that contain gluten, then they are no longer safe to eat. Packaged fries can be coated with wheat (or other starch) to keep them from sticking together. Read labels carefully. You can always hand cut a fresh potato into french fry slices and know your fries are 100 percent free from gluten.

- **Spices:** Natural spices such as sage, garlic, rosemary, and mint are gluten free. Most packaged spices are also free from gluten, but check ingredient labels and manufacturer disclosures carefully as some might be manufactured on lines that also manufacture wheat. Your safest bet is to purchase certified gluten-free spices. All Spicely spices, and some Spice Hunter spices, are certified gluten free.
- **Beans and Lentils:** Beans and lentils are gluten free and a great source of protein. You can buy them fresh inside a bag (soak and prepare them according to instructions) or in a can. Avoid buying beans and lentils from the bulk bins.
- **Cooking Oils:** Cooking oils are free from gluten. I use avocado oil the most because it has a high smoke point and is good for baking and frying at high heat up to 500° F. Canola oil, corn oil, vegetable oil, olive oil, sunflower oil, and coconut oil are all gluten free, but again check the labels to be sure. Some cooking sprays are not gluten free, particularly ones used for baking.

As I thought about what a life without gluten looked like for me, I realized I could still make the vast majority of the meals I've always made. The only difference is that I needed to find gluten-free swaps for some of the ingredients. For example, I could easily enjoy spaghetti and meatballs for dinner as long as I used gluten-free pasta, gluten-free breadcrumbs, and gluten-free pasta sauce. I could still make breaded chicken with gluten-free breadcrumbs, gluten-free lasagna with gluten-free lasagna noodles, gluten-free stir-fry with gluten-free soy sauce or tamari. There are very few meals I can't make with gluten-free ingredients, and I know, with time, you will find this to be true as well.

I also found that this change in my diet served as a launching pad to experiment with new recipes. I was eating at home more often, because it's the safest place to be, so I figured I might as well experiment a bit in the kitchen. I found inspiration by scrolling through Pinterest and looking up recipes from gluten-free bloggers. My most favorite source of inspiration, however, came from published cookbooks that I checked out at my local library. I didn't limit myself to *just* gluten-free cookbooks either, as there are plenty of amazing recipes inside regular cookbooks. I only needed to make a few easy swaps to turn a recipe into a gluten-free feast. Your local library carries a lot of cookbooks, which are available for you to check out. This gives you the opportunity to *try before you buy*. You want to invest only in cookbooks you're going to use and love, so why not sample them first for free?

PLAN, COOK, REPEAT

Learning how to cook is essential to surviving the gluten-free diet. Eating at home, with familiar ingredients, and with your clean, dedicated gluten-free cooking supplies, will always be the safest (and arguably best) way to enjoy eating.

Meal planning is essential to eating well at home and never feeling deprived. When you feel deprived, you end up reaching for *not-so-good-for-you* packaged foods (hello cookies!) out of desperation or hunger. Or, you end up eating basic and boring meals (remember my scrambled egg and apple?) that only make you feel sorry for yourself.

Each week, before you go to the grocery store, write down the meals you plan to eat for the week. Make sure to include meals for breakfast, lunch, dinner and snacking. I often cook an extra portion of dinner to eat for lunch the next day, so don't forget to include planned leftovers in your meal plan.

Meal planning, cooking often, and eating in are all overwhelming at first, but they do get easier with time, especially as you start to learn your way around the kitchen and experiment with new foods. I found figuring out what to eat to be the hardest part of meal planning; I wish someone could have just *told* me what to eat. It's the reason I created my gluten-free meal planning service. I know how hard it is to figure out what to eat day-in and day-out, so I create these meal plans for my clients to take the guesswork out of the process.

Visit goodforyouglutenfree.com/dear-gluten-resources to find a free 7-day meal plan, along with a meal planning template to help you get started.

REBOUND FOODS

As you become better at the gluten-free way of life, you'll realize there are so many commercially available options that make living a gluten-free lifestyle easier. (To clarify, it's never easy to live a gluten-free lifestyle, but it can and will become *easier.*)

Try different foods and brands to find out what swaps work best for you. This "diet" isn't about giving up on eating your favorite foods; rather it's about replacing those foods with gluten-free alternatives. Following are gluten-free brands that you can use in lieu of their gluten-y counterparts. Please note that some of these brands make both gluten-full and gluten-free varieties of their products, so please read labels carefully.

Note: I do not recommend overindulging in packaged foods if you're serious about healing your body, which we will talk about in greater detail in Part II. These are simply brands to get to know and that provide replacements for conventional convenience foods.

- **Baking Mixes:** Betty Crocker, Bob's Red Mill, Chebe, Enjoy Life, Glutino, Immaculate, King Arthur, Krusteaz, liveGfree, Meli's Monster Cookies, Namaste, Pillsbury, Simple Mills, Trader Joe's, ZenSweet
- **Bread:** BFree, Canyon Bakehouse, Ener-G, Glutino, Franz, Kim & Jake's, Kinnikinnick Foods, Little Northern Bakehouse, Schar, The Essential Baking Company, Three Baker's, Trader Joe's, Udi's

- **Breadcrumbs:** 4C Gluten Free Crumbs, Aleia's Gluten-Free Foods, Ian's Natural Foods, Schar, Trader Joe's
- **Cereal:** Barbara's, Cheerios, Chex, liveGfree, Love Grown Foods, Nature's Path, One Degree, Three Wishes Cereal
- **Cookie Dough:** Eat Pastry (GF), Hail Mary, Immaculate, Sweet Loren's (So Delicious makes a GF cookie dough ice cream)
- **Cookies:** Archway, Cybele's Free to Eat, Enjoy Life, Glutenetto, Glutino, Goodie Girl, Homefree, Kinnikinnick Foods, liveGfree, Lucy's Lucky Spoon, Made Good, MI-DEL, Pamela's Products, Partake, Tate's Bake Shop, Trader Joe's, Schar, Sheila G's, Simple Mills, Udi's, WOW Baking Company
- **Crackers:** Absolutely, Blue Diamond, Crunchmaster, Glutino, liveGfree, Mary's Gone Crackers, Milton's, Nabisco's Good Thins, Nairn's, Simple Mills, Trader Joe's, Van's
- **Donuts/Muffins:** Flax 4 Life, Freedom, Katz's, Kinnikinnick, Udi's
- **Flours:** Arrowhead Mills, Bob's Red Mill, Cup 4 Cup, Enjoy Life, GFJules, Honeyville, King Arthur
- **Frozen Entrees/Foods/Misc.:** Amy's, Brazi Bites, Dr. Praeger's, Feel Good Foods, Cappello's, geefree, Hilary's, Ian's Natural Foods, liveGfree, Mikey's, Path of Life, Udi's
- **Granola/Muesli:** Bakery on Main, Bear Naked, Bob's Red Mill, Kind, Made Good, Nature's Path, Purely Elizabeth, Safe + Fair, Seven Sundays, The Toasted Oat, Udi's
- **Mac and Cheese:** Annie's, Banza, Daiya, Pamela's Products, Udi's
- **Oats and Oatmeal:** Bakery on Main, Bob's Red Mill, Glutenfreeda, Nature's Path, Nairn's, One Degree, Purely Elizabeth, Quaker, Three Bears
- **Pancakes/Waffles (frozen):** Birch Benders, Trader Joe's, Van's
- **Pasta:** Ancient Harvest, Banza, Barilla, Cappello's, De Boles, Explore Cuisine, GoGo Quinoa, Jovial, Now

Foods, Ronzoni, RP Pasta, Tinkyada, Tolerant, Trader Joe's, truRoots
- **Pie Crust:** Bob's Red Mill (mix), Kinnikinnick, MI-DEL, Wholly Wholesome
- **Pizza (frozen):** Against the Grain, Cappello's, Cali'flour Foods, Daiya, DiGiorno, Freschetta, Etalia's, liveGfree, Milton's, Real Good Pizza Co., Sabatasso's, Smart Flour Foods, Sonoma Flatbreads, Trader Joe's, Udi's
- **Pretzels:** FitJoy, From the Ground Up, Glutino, liveGfree, Quinn, Snyder's, Snack Factory
- **Puff Pastry:** GeeFree, Katz, Pillsbury, Schar
- **Ramen:** Lotus Foods, Pamela's Products, Thai Kitchen
- **Soy Sauce:** Kikkoman, San-J
- **Tortillas and Wraps:** BFree, liveGfree, Mikey's, Mission, Rudi's, Seite Foods, Udi's

You may have to shop at different grocery stores to find some of these specialty, gluten-free brands, albeit many mainstream stores like Walmart, Target, Kroger, Safeway/Albertsons, Costco, and Sam's Club have come a long way in expanding their gluten-free options.

I prefer to shop at natural- and health-focused grocery stores like Sprouts and Whole Foods. I find they have the best selection of gluten-free name brands. Even discount supermarkets like Trader Joe's and ALDI have their own privately-labeled gluten-free products. If you don't live in a major city where you'll have greater access to gluten-free brands, don't fret. You can have packaged goods delivered to your doorstep thanks to Amazon, Thrive Market, or manufacturer websites. The internet truly has given our community access to gluten-free food wherever we live.

THE BAKING BLUES

While learning to *cook* gluten free meant I had to make a few ingredient swaps here and there, *baking* was an entirely different story. In fact, gluten-free baking can be very humbling and frustrating for even the most experienced of bakers.

The secret to gluten-free baking is to create a gluten-free flour blend, which consists of a variety of flours, starches, and gums (typically xanthan and guar gum). Doing this will ensure your flour mixture mimics the texture of wheat flour, and your recipe won't fall flat or taste gritty. You cannot simply swap plain rice flour on a 1:1 basis for wheat flour. It won't work.

I recommend using commercially available 1:1 gluten-free flour blends and finding recipes that call for 1:1 gluten-free flour blends. For example, if your recipe calls for one cup of wheat flour, you simply swap it for one cup of a 1:1 gluten-free flour blend. Here are some of the commercially available 1:1 blends available on the market (listed in alphabetical order):

- Better Batter All-Purpose Flour Mix
- Bob's Red Mill 1-to-1 Gluten-Free Flour Blend
- Cup-4-Cup Gluten-Free Flour
- GFJules All-Purpose Gluten-Free Flour
- Great Value All-Purpose Gluten-Free Flour (Walmart brand)
- King Arthur Gluten-Free All-Purpose Flour
- Krusteaz Gluten-Free All-Purpose Flour
- Namaste Perfect Flour Blend
- Pamela's Gluten-Free All-Purpose Flour
- Pillsbury Gluten-Free Multi-Purpose Flour Blend
- Ryze Gluten-Free Flour Mix

Keep in mind that some of these gluten-free flour blends contain dairy or corn, so check ingredient labels if you're avoiding other ingredients besides gluten. As you become more adventurous, you can try baking with grain-free flours such as almond flour, chickpea flour, quinoa flour and coconut flour. Be aware, however, that these flours are not meant to be used as 1:1 swap with wheat flour in your recipes. You'll want to find recipes specifically using these flours to get started.

Almond flour is my preferred grain-free flour as it doesn't have a strong, nutty taste like other nut flours and coconut flour. It makes baked goods moist and works well in cakes and cookies. Almond flour, however, has a high fat content so you'll need to adjust the amount of oil or butter (fats) in your recipes to prevent your baked goods from being greasy.

Cassava flour is another grain-free flour that can be used as a 1:1 swap with wheat flour when measured by weight vs. volume. You'll need a kitchen scale to bake with cassava flour, and I highly recommend investing in one, which will cost you less than $20. Let's say your recipe calls for 280 grams of wheat flour, then you'd use 280 grams of cassava flour instead. I find the texture of cassava flour in baked goods to be good, and have tested it in cakes, cookies and tortillas with great success. It can be a useful flour for anyone who is looking for a grain-free, nut-free, single ingredient 1:1 flour option. Bob's Red Mill, Iya Foods, Otto's Naturals, and Pamela's make and sell cassava flour that works well for grain-free baking.

CHAPTER 5
EASING INTO EATING OUT

"One cannot think well, love well, sleep
well, if one has not dined well."

– Virginia Woolf

Eating out post-breakup is extremely challenging, especially at first. Gluten is everywhere, and restaurants are riddled with reminders of your ex – i.e., the foods you can no longer eat. In fact, eating out can be quite the humbling and depressing experience at first, and you'll soon learn that many of your favorite restaurants and beloved foods, like pizza and sandwiches, are now off limits, with a few exceptions.

The truth is, while I eat the vast majority of my meals at home because it's the safest place to eat, I love eating out and do so a few times each week. I enjoy trying new restaurants, going out to celebrate happy occasions with friends and family, and not having to cook every night.

I know a lot of people with celiac disease and gluten sensitivities who are scared and anxious to eat out at all. I get it. There's nothing worse than getting sick and having to sit on the toilet for a while in the middle of a romantic date or family outing.

The truth is, eating out sans gluten is doable, and you should continue to enjoy eating out if it is a normal part of your lifestyle. There is no need to give it up altogether or commit social suicide, especially if eating out is your jam.

Mind you, I do not take eating out lightly. I take a lot of precautions to do it right and as safely as possible. There will always be an inherent risk no matter how many precautions you take. One study even found gluten in 32 percent of restaurant dishes specified as "gluten free."[48] That said, there are steps you can take to minimize the potential risk of gluten exposure, all of which I will detail in this chapter.

WHY IS IT SO HARD?

I'm not looking for restaurants to roll out the red carpet for me, nor cater to my every wish; rather, I simply want to be able to eat something safe, be with my friends, and not feel like a social pariah.

That's why I'm truly astonished by how hard someone with celiac disease or gluten sensitivity has to work to be taken seriously by restaurant staff these days. I try to understand it, though. Servers have to deal with people and all their idiosyncrasies and the myriad of food allergies prevalent today. They are often serving people who are not serious about eating gluten free, which creates confusion and hypocrisy at the dinner table. For example, a not-so-serious gluten-free diner may order a gluten-free meal and a beer, or ask for their soup order to be gluten free but still want the baguette that comes with it. Confusing indeed!

At first I thought these stories of people ordering gluten-free meals along with gluten-y beer were urban legend, but then it happened right before my eyes. I went out to lunch with a few girlfriends once; some of us were eating gluten free and some weren't. We ordered a few dishes, family-style, to share. Half of the dishes were gluten free, half were not. When the order came, I watched one of my gluten-free girlfriends take what she said was "just a little taste" of one of the dishes that contained gluten.

"It's not gluten free!" I urgently warned, but she responded by quipping, "A little bit of gluten doesn't bother me."

I was livid. How could a person say she's gluten free, make a fuss about it to the waiter, and then sit there and eat "just a bite" of gluten?

What's even more frustrating are those individuals who should be fully committed to the gluten-free diet, like those with diagnosed celiac disease or gluten sensitivity, but who aren't following the diet to a T nor taking it seriously. Such individuals make it hard for those of us with medically-necessary dietary restrictions, and those who are resolute about eating strictly gluten free, to be taken seriously by restaurant staff.

This is why, when eating out, you have to advocate firmly for yourself and block out what others might or might not be doing or thinking when ordering gluten-free meals. When ordering food at a restaurant, you must be confident, kind, and assertive when speaking with those preparing your food. This is the only way they'll know you're serious about your diet, and it will encourage them to take the proper precautions in preparing your food. In other words, the more firmly you communicate your needs, the more the restaurant staff will know you mean business. I'll talk about how to convey the seriousness of your diet a bit later in this chapter.

IDENTIFYING SAFE RESTAURANTS

Many restaurants offer gluten-free options today, which is great news for our community. However, not all of them are doing gluten free right. Let's talk about where you can eat, and how you can sniff out the good from the bad.

The best way to find restaurants when you first break up with gluten is to search for them online. Local gluten-free bloggers can provide excellent information about restaurant finds in your city. There are also several excellent apps that crowdsource gluten-free restaurant information, such as the Find Me Gluten-Free app.

Another option is to ask others where they eat. You probably have a friend who is already eating gluten free and can help you get started with a good list.

CHAIN RESTAURANTS WITH GLUTEN-FREE OPTIONS*:

I have not independently verified all the restaurants on this list. The best and most current information will always be at each individual restaurant.

- Applebee's
- Bonefish Grill
- Boston Market
- California Pizza Kitchen
- Caribou Coffee
- Carrabba's Italian Grill
- Cheesecake Factory
- Chick-fil-a
- Chili's
- Chipotle
- First Watch
- Five Guys
- Honest Burger (UK)
- In-n-Out Burger
- Jersey Mike's
- Legal Sea Foods
- Maggiano's
- Melting Pot
- Modern Market
- Noodles and Company
- The Original Pancake House (select locations)
- Olive Garden
- Outback Steakhouse
- Panera

- Pappadeaux Seafood Kitchen
- Pei Wei
- PF Chang's
- Pizza Hut (select locations)
- Qdoba
- Red Robin
- Ruby Tuesday
- Shake Shack
- Starbucks
- Wendy's

For a full list of chain restaurants with gluten-free options, visit goodforyouglutenfree.com/dear-gluten-resources.

*Just because a restaurant is listed does not mean it does gluten free right; it only means it offers gluten-free options.

Many chain restaurants have good protocols in place to help you navigate around gluten. As you become more adventurous, you can look for restaurants off the beaten path. There are plenty of small, local restaurants that do gluten free right.

Before visiting a restaurant for the first time, research its menu online and call them. Don't expect a restaurant to cater to you the minute you walk in the door if you haven't taken the time to call ahead and learn more about how they handle gluten-free requests. I once called a restaurant that my extended family suggested for brunch. The woman I spoke to said in not so many words, "Don't eat here if you can't eat gluten." Her brutal honesty hurt me, but at the same time, she also saved me from eating there and getting sick. I was glad to have the opportunity to take my business elsewhere.

On the other side of the coin, I have enjoyed many comforting conversations with restaurant staff. Many restaurants have been able to accommodate me with plenty of options. Some, when I've called ahead and given them notice that I'm coming, have even offered to make me a special dish or dessert. Sweet! This is a restaurant that wants my business and one where I will sing its praises time and time again.

This kindness was extended to me when traveling abroad. A hotel in Amsterdam didn't know I needed a gluten-free breakfast until I showed up at the breakfast buffet during the first morning of my stay. The staff was pleasant and scrambled to make me a great meal. The waiter asked me how long I was staying; I told him one more night. The next morning the staff had warm, gluten-free croissants and muffins waiting for me. They had also prepared a breakfast feast for me, a kindness I will never forget.

Most restaurants do not allow outside food in their establishments; this means you cannot bring your own meal. I once brought my own sandwich into a restaurant because, when I had called ahead, they could not assure me a safe meal. The group I was with insisted on going there, so I was stuck. When I started eating my sandwich, the manager came over to my table and told me no outside food was allowed. While I respected his rule, I explained that his staff said they could not accommodate me, and I wanted to enjoy lunch with my friends. It was an awkward situation. Instead of making a scene, I simply tucked the sandwich into my purse and sipped on fresh water while everyone else ate their lunch. I could enjoy my sandwich later.

I've since learned that the Americans with Disabilities Act (ADA) states that you may bring your own food into a restaurant that is unable to accommodate your dietary needs. It's a law that has actually been tested. A train tour operator in New Hampshire refused to allow a customer to bring her own allergy-friendly food onboard. When challenged by the ADA, the train tour operator revised its policies to make "alternate dietary selections available to all customers upon 24 hours' notice."[49]

The ADA, however, cannot force a restaurant to provide you with gluten-free food because it would require restaurants to meet every single food accommodation imaginable. Because bringing your own food is awkward at best (I don't suggest doing it), I recommend finding restaurants willing to accommodate you. There's nothing more powerful than speaking with your wallet.

Today, if I must go to a restaurant that cannot accommodate me, which typically happens when I'm a part of a tour or large group where I have no say in where we're going, I simply eat ahead of time, enjoy a drink while I'm there, and relish the time with my friends. If questioned by the manager or waitstaff why I'm not eating, I graciously explain that I called ahead and the manager told me there is nothing safe for me to eat here.

The good news is that your friends and family will often defer to you when it comes to picking the restaurant. The last thing they want to do is eat in front of you while you just sit there. Because I'm often asked to pick the restaurant, I keep a running list of restaurants I like and restaurants people recommend to me in the Notes app on my phone. I'm always ready with a suggestion when asked.

WHAT THE HECK IS A *GLUTEN-CONSCIOUS* MENU?

As you begin to eat out more, you'll start to see menus that say they're everything but a "gluten-free menu," including *gluten sensitive, gluten intolerant, gluten-free friendly* or *gluten conscious* menus. Very few restaurants will have a "gluten-free" or "celiac-safe" menu, mainly because they can't (or don't want to) guarantee your meal will be free from gluten. This is a restaurant's way of legally getting out of providing you a safe meal, while cashing in on the gluten-free trend.

I get it. It's hard for a restaurant to guarantee a safe meal for someone who cannot eat even a crumb of gluten. A busy restaurant handles a lot of gluten in its kitchen and doesn't want to make you sick nor be responsible if you get sick. They want to be able to say, "We told you we couldn't guarantee a gluten-free meal, as evident by our *gluten-sensitive menu*. If you want to eat here, do so at your own risk."

Further, if a restaurant claims its food is "gluten free," it must meet the FDA gluten-free labeling guidelines with food that contains no more than 20 ppm of gluten. I don't know any restaurant that has the ability to test dishes for gluten before serving it to a diner. Making a "gluten-free" claim, as you can see, is not a prudent thing for a restaurant to do.

So that leads me back to the *gluten-sensitive* or *gluten-conscious* menu, and understanding whether it's safe for you to eat at that particular restaurant. Personally, I'm comfortable eating at restaurants with menus that come with all sorts of clever *gluten-something* names. That said, I'm extremely cautious about what I will order and eat. I always express the seriousness of my diet, and I ask a lot of questions to make sure I get the safest meal possible. Is it a risk to eat out? Absolutely. And this risk is inherent whether it says *gluten-free* or *gluten-sensitive* at the top of the menu.

Along with the *gluten-something* menu, you will typically find a disclaimer either on the menu, or recited to you out loud by your server. A restaurant's disclaimer goes something like, "While we have foods that do not contain gluten, we cannot guarantee your meal will be gluten free because we do not have a dedicated gluten-free kitchen." When I'm faced with this disclaimer, I kindly respond by asking the staff to change gloves, wipe down surfaces, and do their best to keep my food separate from gluten. I ask them to point me to the safest, least risky dish on the menu, and thank them for their attention and consideration in preparing a safe meal for me so I can enjoy this time with my friends. I choose my words carefully, offering subtle hints that remind them that I'm a human being wanting to enjoy a meal out with my family and friends.

I've often found it frustrating that restaurants are using all these confusing terms in order to cash in on the gluten-free trend, but do little to make their food safe for people with celiac disease or gluten sensitivities. If you're going to offer any sort of gluten-free (or gluten-sensitive or gluten-conscious) food without making a sincere effort to provide a safe meal for those of us who need it most, then don't do it in the first place. Panera, for example, makes gluten-conscious cookies that it places right next to the gluten-y cookies in its bakery display case. The restaurant chain makes no attempt to create a safe space for its gluten-free baked goods. Papa John's and Domino's Pizza both make gluten-free pizza crust, yet both restaurants say they do not recommend their gluten-free pizza for people with celiac disease. Ho hum.

DECODING WHAT'S *REALLY* IN YOUR FOOD?

When eating out, you'll want to make sure the person preparing your food knows what he or she is doing. This is why it's important to ask your server a lot of questions. You can usually sniff out an inexperienced server and/or restaurant pretty quickly. When this happens, ask to speak with the manager or chef. You need someone to give you confidence that you will get a safe meal. As a rule of thumb, never assume a restaurateur, caterer, server, or chef knows gluten free like you.

Specifically, ask your server in-depth questions related to the following foods and preparation methods:

The Deep Fryer: If you want to order something that is deep fried, like french fries, you must first ask if the fryer used to cook your fries is a dedicated gluten-free fryer. If it is, then you're okay, if not, nix fries from your order. While an innocent french fry is naturally gluten free as it's made from potatoes, if it's placed in the same boiling oil as breaded chicken nuggets, then bits of the gluten from the nuggets will seep into or on your fries. Keep in mind that some restaurants will claim their fries are gluten free even if they are cooked in a shared fryer. When in doubt, avoid all fried foods when eating out. It's just not worth it.

Following are the most common deep-fried foods you must be suspicious of gluten cross-contamination when eating out:

- Breaded Chinese food dishes (sesame chicken, sweet and sour chicken)
- Calamari
- Chicken fingers

- Chicken wings
- Corn dogs
- Corn or tortilla chips
- Donuts
- Egg rolls
- Falafel
- Fish sticks
- French fries
- Fried appetizers
- Fried chicken
- Fritters
- Onion rings
- Samosas
- Tempura
- Wontons

The Griddle or Grill: Your gluten-free pancakes made with gluten-free flour might be cooked on the same surface used to cook gluten-y pancakes. Before ordering pancakes, ask how they're cooked, and inquire if it's possible for them to cook your gluten-free pancakes in a clean pan vs. the shared griddle.

The Toaster: There is a slim chance that a restaurant will have a dedicated gluten-free toaster, so this means the gluten-free toast they're offering is, you guessed it, being toasted in the same device used to toast wheat bread. I never order gluten-free toast; I always ask if they can substitute fresh fruit for the toast instead.

The Waffle Iron: Cooking gluten-free waffle batter in a waffle iron used to cook batter with wheat flour ensures your waffle will contain gluten. No thanks. Waffles are off limits.

The Pasta Water: Most restaurants are good about cooking their gluten-free pasta in separate water, handling it with separate tongs, and draining it with separate colanders, but alas, some are not and mistakes can happen. If you order pasta, ask lots of questions. I rarely order pasta anymore. It's just too risky. I just enjoy pasta at home.

How to Order

I cannot emphasize enough how important it is that you disclose to your server (or whoever is preparing your meal) that you cannot eat gluten. Don't just order a gluten-free meal or order a meal and assume it's gluten free. It's important that you tell your server, upfront, something like, "I cannot eat gluten, and I'm serious about it. Gluten makes me really sick. Can you help me get a safe meal?" The firmer you are about your request, the more likely your server will take your order seriously. If you don't disclose the seriousness of your request, don't expect your server to take you seriously.

Gluten is not an "allergen" and, therefore, you cannot be allergic to gluten. However, when dealing with restaurant staff, using the word "allergy" will alert the staff, in their own language, about the seriousness of your order. Your server probably won't understand what you're talking about if you say, "I have an autoimmune disease where gluten triggers my immune system to attack my body." Similarly, only some servers will take you seriously if you say, "I have gluten sensitivity." Instead of dancing around the issue, use the word "allergy" or request "allergy prep" as restaurants know and understand what to do when someone requests it. When you request allergy prep, most restaurants will take precautions such as washing their hands, changing gloves, wiping down surfaces, and preparing your meal using a clean pan. Of course, you may have to ask them if they take these precautions and insist they do so for you.

When I visit Chipotle, for example, I tell the server I have a "gluten allergy" and ask if he (or she) will wash his hands and change his gloves. I then ask that person to stay with me from start to finish on the assembly line. I'm fine with him scooping rice, meat and salsas into my burrito bowl, but when we get to the cheese and lettuce, I ask him to pull those items from fresh containers in the back, and he always happily obliges. The reason I do this is because, if you examine the Chipotle serving line, you'll see that everything is scooped with utensils, except for the cheese and lettuce. Those items are scooped by hand, and those hands that have touched gluten and likely transferred gluten-y bits onto the cheese and lettuce.

Although it's tempting to order pizza, pasta, or waffles at restaurants, the truth is it's not generally safe to eat these foods outside the confines of your home. It's just too risky; and if you're serious about eating gluten free, don't take this risk. Restaurant pizza is almost never safe. While a pizza place might have a gluten-free crust, they still use shared ingredients, shared utensils, and shared surfaces. They also might use the same peel – a shovel-like tool used to slide the pizza in and out of the oven – and they also might place the gluten-free pizza on the same spot inside the oven where gluten-y pizza has been cooked. That said, gluten-free pizza restaurants do exist and some really work hard to accommodate gluten-free eaters. When you find a pizza restaurant that knows what it's doing, treasure it. Order from it regularly and speak loudly with your wallet to help it stay in business.

The way I minimize my risk of getting sick and compromising my health when eating out is that I try to always order naturally gluten-free items such as a bunless burger, baked salmon, roasted chicken, a fresh salad, a veggie-loaded omelet, and/or a baked potato. These items are least likely to contain and/or come in contact with gluten during preparation.

Further, to ensure a safe dining experience from start to finish, always confirm with your server that the dish placed before you is the gluten-free meal you ordered. A lot can become tangled up in the kitchen between the time you place your order and when a meal is placed before you. I suggest you ask your server "how" they know it's the gluten-free dish. They usually will be able to tell you how they know for sure that the dish is gluten free.

Also, look for visual clues that will help you decode if the meal placed before you is gluten free. Pei Wei, for example, uses different colored bowls/plates to serve its gluten-free items. Red Robin and First Watch restaurants put a toothpick in their gluten-free dishes to ensure communication is clear from the kitchen to the server and ultimately to the customer.

NAVIGATING BUFFETS

Unfortunately, buffets are notoriously known for cross-contamination. Even if something is labeled gluten free on a buffet, it doesn't mean it's actually gluten free by the time it makes it on your plate. Buffets, for all intents and purposes, are not a pretty site when you eat gluten free.

Do yourself a favor. The next time you're at a buffet, do a little people watching; you'll see all sorts of red flags such as:

- Shared utensils being used to scoop different dishes. The spoon for the rice has somehow made its way into the stuffing tray.
- Food dripping everywhere as people scoop heaping portions on their plates. It's always an unsettling site when I see a stray crouton floating in the Italian dressing.
- The utensils used to scoop a gluten-free dish, like meat sauce, coming in contact with a gluten-y dish like pasta when scooped onto a plate.

If you must eat at a buffet, here are a few tips to eating as safely as possible. Even someone as strict as I am has been able to successfully navigate a buffet or two in my lifetime.

Assess the Situation: Take note of all potential cross-contamination risks. Sometimes the gluten-free items are strategically placed far away from the breads and gluten-y items. An Indian buffet in Denver offers a nearly 100 percent gluten-free lunch buffet and the only non-GF item on the buffet is the naan (bread). The owner conscientiously has placed the naan at the end of the buffet line so people take it last and, thereby, don't contaminate the otherwise gluten-free buffet.

Speak With the Manager: Explain that you need a safe, gluten-free meal and ask if he or she can show you which items you can and cannot eat. If the buffet looks cross-contaminated beyond what you feel comfortable eating, let the manager know and ask if it would be possible to take from freshly prepared foods that haven't been placed on the buffet table yet. Some managers will even make you a special meal, if requested. The chef at the Wynn Buffet in Las Vegas made me all fresh food. I ate so much that day!

Don't Eat: When all else fails, don't eat. Just enjoy a few snacks from your purse or coat pocket and know you'll get to eat later when it's safe to do so. No buffet is worth the risk, and some buffets are just too difficult for anyone on a gluten-free diet to bear.

TESTING YOUR FOOD

In addition to looking for visual signs of gluten in every dish you eat, you can also test your food for hidden gluten using a portable gluten detecting device called the Nima Sensor. (Please note that Medline Industries, a medical device company, purchased the Nima Sensor in 2020 and the fate of the device is unknown as of publication.)

To test your food for hidden gluten, put a small piece of your food into the single-use test capsule, place the capsule inside the sensor, and then press the start button. In about 1-2 minutes, the sensor will tell you it has detected gluten by displaying a "gluten found" message or by displaying a smiley face if it does not find gluten.

This gadget is perfect when I'm thinking this bun placed before me looks too good to be gluten free, or when my waiter tells me the french fries are gluten free but I see many fried items on the menu. The Nima Sensor is 96.9 percent accurate at detecting gluten at 20 ppm or higher.[50]

Unfortunately, nothing is foolproof, not even the Nima Sensor. It cannot detect gluten in fermented foods like soy sauce and alcohol because, in these cases, the fermentation process breaks down the gluten particle into tiny, undetectable bits. This is why you must ensure only gluten-free ingredients are used to prepare your dish whether or not you test it with your sensor. The device also only tests a small portion of your food, not the entire dish, so you can't know for sure if other parts of your dish have been exposed to cross-contamination. A testing device is not a substitute for asking questions, conveying the seriousness of your request, and taking all the steps necessary to ensure you wind up with a safe meal. I encourage you to do more research on this gadget before investing in it. You can learn more about it at: goodforyouglutenfree.com/nima-sensor.

DINING WHILE TRAVELING

Eating gluten free while traveling is another challenge you'll face if you have celiac disease or gluten sensitivity. There are some countries that get it right, and some that remain clueless about gluten disorders.

I personally found great success eating out gluten free in London, Tel Aviv, and Amsterdam, albeit I struggled a bit in Paris. I hear countries like Italy and Finland offer amazing gluten-free options, too. Of course, when traveling, always bring along emergency food, look up grocery stores near where you're staying, and book a room with a kitchenette so you can store and prepare simple meals without being dependent on restaurants. I also recommend bringing along a gluten-free dining card in the language of the country you're visiting. (Google "Gluten-Free Dining Card + Spanish," for example). The dining card will convey your needs in the country's language to help ensure you get a safe meal.

I have found that cruise ships are particularly friendly to people with food allergies. You just need to know how to navigate them properly. In my experience, it's key to discuss your food allergy with the head waiter and pre-order meals as much as possible. It can be a bit tricky on Day 1 because the staff is just getting to know you; but if you continually order your meals ahead of time, you should be in great shape. The ship staff will also pack a lunch for you, upon request, so you have food during your off-ship excursions. You can read more about my strategies for cruising while gluten free in this article: goodforyouglutenfree. com/your-ultimate-gluten-free-cruise-survival-guide/.

Another great location for gluten-free dining is Disneyworld and Disneyland. Disney handles food allergies with ease and never makes you feel like a second-class diner. Disney staff is well trained in handling food allergies and offers plenty of options in all its parks.

ATTENDING SPECIAL EVENTS

Before attending any special event, it's important to discuss your food needs with the host. Some people find it hard to approach the host, such as a bride or conference organizer, to ask for a gluten-free meal; but I assure you, it's okay to do – and it's the right thing to do. The host is paying for you to eat, and the caterer will most likely be happy to accommodate you and include the cost of your meal in his or her service.

It's always nice when the reply card inside the invitation asks for special dietary requests. If it doesn't, write your request on the card and follow up with the host. You can say something like, "I don't want to create more work for you, but if it's possible for me to get a gluten-free meal, I'd like that. I'm happy to coordinate with your caterer." It's always a plus when you have direct access to the caterer. If the caterer cannot accommodate you, simply bring your own food and make sure the host doesn't pay for a meal you can't eat!

The same goes for conferences and business luncheons. These events are a bit different because more likely than not, you're paying an attendance fee and that fee includes the cost of your meals. I go to events all the time and always ask for a gluten-free meal. The key is to plan in advance and not spring your request on the host the day of the event; rather, email the event host a few months or weeks before the event and tell them your dietary needs. More likely than not they will be able to accommodate with a little notice. If not, tell them you're happy to bring your own food but would like a refund for the meal portion of your ticket. There's no sense in paying for a meal you *can't* eat, especially when you have to shell out money to buy a meal you *can* eat.

These moments can test your bravery, but they are a necessary step to living with a gluten disorder. I've become used to doing this, and I promise it gets easier with time. Now I don't hesitate; I just do it!

EATING OUT CHECKLIST

The following checklist will walk you through the eating out process:

- ☐ Properly vet a restaurant before visiting. Call ahead if needed.
- ☐ Convey the seriousness of your dietary needs to your server.
- ☐ Ask questions to gauge your server's understanding of gluten. Elevate your request to the manager or chef if your server is not familiar with gluten, does not understand your request, or does not take you seriously.
- ☐ Request "allergy prep." Ask that the staff wash hands and change gloves before preparing your meal.
- ☐ Confirm that the meal placed before you is gluten free.
- ☐ Test your meal for hidden gluten (optional).
- ☐ Be gracious and thank the staff for the extra assistance in preparing a safe meal for you. Leave a tip that reflects your appreciation.
- ☐ Leave an honest review on an app or online dining site to share your experiences and help make the world better for the next gluten-free diner. Remember to speak with your wallet and frequent restaurants that do gluten free well.

Chapter 6
Looking Good & Feeling Good Post Breakup

"Have nothing in your house that you do not know to be useful or believe to be beautiful."

– William Morris

Unfortunately, gluten isn't found only in the food you eat. It may be lurking inside your medicine cabinets and vanities. Just as your ex may have left behind his toothbrush or comb, it's time to make sure no gluten crumbs are lurking inside your medicine cabinet and bathroom. It's time to evict gluten – and all traces of it – from all facets of your life, for good.

Gluten in Medications

While the food industry follows specific guidelines related to how much gluten it can include in a product in order for it to be labeled "gluten free" (no more than 20 parts per million), there are no guidelines for pharmaceuticals. This means a pill meant to help you feel better might actually be making you sick, or potentially worse, you may forgo taking an important medication because you're terrified of getting glutened – ack!

A 2019 study published in *Science Translational Medicine* found that gluten may be found in more medications than we realize.[51] Researchers referenced a study where 18 percent of drug manufacturers admit that their medications contained gluten as an inactive ingredient. Of course, the labels rarely say "gluten" or "wheat"; instead, most drug manufacturers use the term "starch."

How do you know if the drug you're about to take to relieve your symptoms isn't one of the 18 percent of drugs that contain gluten?

I decided to look to the FDA for answers. In its report, "Gluten in Drug Products and Associated Labeling Recommendations Guidance for Industry," the FDA says that most medications don't contain gluten (wheat, barley or rye), and those that do have only trace amounts that the FDA says are "safe" for someone with celiac disease to ingest.[52] The FDA adds that barley and rye are either used "rarely or not at all" in the production of medications.

All this sounds encouraging, but what about the study where 18 percent of drug manufacturers said that their medications contain gluten? How can you be absolutely certain that your medication is not among the 18 percent?

While we may not know now, the good news is that the FDA is currently pressuring pharmaceutical companies to voluntarily disclose gluten – and other allergens – in medications, inclusive of both oral medications and topical medications applied in or around the mouth. This is why you might soon be seeing drug labels with allergen statements such as, *"Contains no ingredient made from a gluten-containing grain (wheat, barley, or rye)."*

I find the game of *figuring out what ingredients are inside the medicine cabinet* extremely frustrating. Take for example a drug used by millions of people every day: Benadryl. I had heard from a member of the gluten-free community that Benadryl was not gluten free, so I tried to independently verify this information with Johnson & Johnson. I received the most disappointing reply. A representative wrote to me, "Sadly, we do not have any information on whether our BENADRYL® Allergy Tablets have gluten or not."[53] Yes, friends, Johnson & Johnson, a multi-billion-dollar company, doesn't know what ingredients are in its products! While it's encouraging that the FDA is taking steps to inform consumers about the ingredients in medications, the agency needs to do more to persuade or mandate pharmaceutical companies to disclose ingredients and allergens. That is the only way the FDA can truly protect the celiac and gluten sensitive communities.

WHAT'S A GLUTEN-FREE PERSON TO DO?

If you need to take (or are already taking) an over-the-counter or prescription drug, there are a few steps you can follow to understand if your medication is safe or not.

Inspect the Label: Many drug manufacturers are currently making voluntary allergen disclosures. Look under the "description" and "inactive ingredient" sections. If you see the word "starch," take pause. If you are suspicious the drug contains gluten, look at the generic version or other brands to see if you can find something similar more clearly labeled.

Ask the Pharmacist: While most pharmacists are in the dark regarding what is or isn't gluten free, it's good to have a conversation with them to see if they *might* know. The more we ask and demand answers, the more the pharmacist (hopefully) will demand answers from drug manufacturers as a result. Perhaps pharmacists can help champion change as well, especially if they're getting the question, "Is it gluten free?" over and over again.

Check pillbox.nlm.nih.gov: If the ingredients are unclear or not disclosed on the label, search for the name of that drug on Pillbox. Pillbox is a site published by the National Institutes of Health's National Library of Medicine. It can be *somewhat* helpful as you try to decode ingredients in medications.

The best way to use Pillbox is to enter a keyword(s). I searched for "wheat" and "gluten" to see if any medications popped up. Here's what I found:

- 20 medications cite wheat as an inactive ingredient
- 1 medication contains the keyword "gluten"
- 14,009 contain the keyword "starch"

As you can see, the vast majority of medications, according to Pillbox, do not contain wheat or gluten; however, a large number of them contain "starch," which could come from any number of ingredients including but not limited to wheat, corn, potato, or tapioca starch. Some of the medications listed on Pillbox indicate the type of starch used, such as cornstarch or potato starch, while other medication labels don't.

Contact the Manufacturer: It's worth trying to see if you can get a clear-cut answer about a specific medication directly from the manufacturer. Unfortunately, many times you will receive a reply like the one Johnson & Johnson sent me, or a wishy-washy reply that offers little comfort. These replies look something like this: "*Our product does not contain gluten ingredients, but we cannot guarantee the product is gluten free.*" Don't give up. It's important that we continue to ask drug manufacturers for this kind of information. The more we ask, the more they will have to answer us and the more it will encourage them to be proactive in labeling (so we don't have to keep asking).

Research Online: The internet is a helpful place for crowd-sourcing information; however, not everything you read or see on the internet is accurate or truthful. It can, however, be useful in seeing how others have approached your same situation; I personally find crowdsourcing such information to be more helpful than many doctors or pharmacists when it comes to decoding gluten in medications.

In the meantime, continue to ask the FDA to create mandatory labeling laws and demand more transparency from drug manufacturers. Keep asking the questions and making noise. Change is coming.

At the Dentist

A few years ago, my dentist wanted to take a mold of my mouth. She began mixing some flour-like substance with water. I paused and asked, "Does that have gluten in it?" She went to check (before putting the substance in my mouth), and came back with a clear answer. "Good news! No gluten, it's just chemicals," she joked. I was relieved, sort of.

When in the dentist chair, make sure all the products your dentist or hygienist puts in your mouth are indeed free from gluten. Yes, even your dentist needs to know you can't eat gluten.

Along the same lines, you may be relieved to know that most mainstream toothpaste brands are also free from gluten. While you should scrutinize the ingredients of any brand before using it, as manufacturing processes and ingredients can change, Arm & Hammer, Aquafresh, Biotene, Crest, Colgate, Oral-B, Sensodyne, and Tom's of Maine are brands that carry products free from gluten.

Gluten in Beauty Products

Current research says that gluten cannot be absorbed into the skin, meaning that you can touch gluten and be okay. If, for example, gluten is an ingredient in your body lotion, it cannot cause an autoimmune reaction (celiac) or inflammation (gluten sensitivity). Hopefully, researchers will continue to study this to make sure it is true. Many drugs are applied topically and absorbed by the skin. Birth control, for example, can be administered through a patch, and pain relief creams are absorbed by your skin. Even nicotine can be absorbed into your body via a patch. That said, current research reports that gluten does no harm when touched or applied to the skin. (Please note that people with a wheat allergy can have an allergic reaction just by touching wheat or products that contain wheat.)

It doesn't take a rocket scientist to know that what we touch may find its way into our mouths. Makeup applied to your face can rub off on your hands, then your hands touch your food, and then, well, you get glutened. Or let's say you're applying blush and the dust lands on your lips. You lick your lips and, boom, gluten has just made its way into your intestines!

On top of that, after I began to follow the gluten-free diet, I started to get this annoying and recurring pink eye. At the time, I hadn't researched any of my makeup for gluten; however, I began to wonder if gluten could be the root cause of my recurring eye infections. I began to research all of my makeup, one-by-one, until I realized my mascara contained wheat germ oil. I immediately switched to a gluten-free brand, used the drops one last time to clear my pink eye, and, as predicted, the pink eye went away and never came back.

It is then that I went on a mission to clear my bathroom of gluten and realized that most mainstream brands do not offer gluten-free products. Unfortunately, when you inquire with manufacturers about gluten in their products, you'll find that some do, some don't, some can't guarantee this or that, and most won't make promises or guarantees. It's unfortunate in today's tech-savvy world that big companies don't know or won't confirm what ingredients they're putting in their products. Again, my hope is that with time, and as more consumers speak with their wallets, we'll see change.

HOW TO PROTECT YOURSELF

The best way to protect yourself is to become an educated consumer. Here are some specific tips to help your gluten-free beauty shine:

Beware of Questionable Ingredients: When assessing a beauty product for gluten, obviously avoid products that contain wheat, barley, rye, or oats (unless oats are noted as gluten free). However, there are other *not-so-obvious* gluten-containing ingredients hidden in many cosmetics, including but not limited to:

- Avena sativa (oat bran)
- Colloidal oatmeal
- Hordeum vulgare (barley)

- Secale cereale (rye seed)
- Tocopherols (may be derived from wheat)
- Tocotrienols (may be derived from wheat)
- Vitamin E (most commonly derived from wheat, but can be derived from soybean or other sources)
- Triticum vulgare (wheat bran or wheat germ oil)

Make Sure All Lip Products Are Gluten Free: This includes lipsticks, lip glosses, and lip balms. While you don't *eat* your lip balm, per se, it does come in contact with your mouth, so naturally you may ingest it.

I researched many of the *mainstream* brands of lip balms and found a mixed bag of confusing information. For example, Burt's Bees, one of the leading "natural" lip balm manufacturers, states the following on its website:

"We cannot provide a list of Burt's Bees products that are safe for use with your [gluten] allergy because our products may have been manufactured on a shared line with products containing gluten, or raw materials used in our products may have been processed in a facility that also processes products containing gluten. Therefore, we are unable to state that any Burt's Bees products are 'gluten free.'"

Based on this information, I am wary about using Burt's Bees products even though, after reviewing the Burt's Bees lip balm ingredient list, I did not see any gluten-containing ingredients. If you're concerned whether your mainstream lip balm is gluten free, read my full report at: goodforyouglutenfree.com/lip-balm-gluten-free.

Use Only Gluten-Free Labeled Products: It's always wise to err on the side of caution when choosing beauty products to slather over your face and body. However, what you'll find is that brands have some products that contain gluten and some that do not. It's so confusing! The good news is that the following brands label their products as "gluten free," and some are even certified gluten free (when noted). Always carefully read labels on individual products.

- Andalou (all products are gluten free and third-party tested by the Food Allergy and Resource Program, according to the Andalou website)
- Arbonne's (the vast majority of beauty products are certified gluten free)
- Badger (lip balms are certified gluten free)
- Derma E (all products are gluten free)
- Dr. Bronner's (all products are gluten free)
- EO and Everyone brand products (all products are certified gluten free)
- EOS (lip balms are gluten free)
- Gabriel Cosmetics (all products are certified gluten free)
- Kiss My Face (all products are gluten free)
- Mineral Fusion (all products are gluten free)
- MyChelle (all products are certified gluten free)
- Nourish Organic (all products are gluten free)
- Pangea Organics (all products are gluten free)
- Red Apple Lipstick (all products are certified gluten free)
- Seaweed Bath Co. (all products are gluten free)
- Thayer's Natural Remedies (all products are gluten free)
- Tom's of Maine (all products are gluten free)

You can find a lot of these products at Whole Foods, Sprouts, and/or your local natural grocery store while others you'll need to shop for online. I know firsthand the hardship involved with switching up my makeup brand and beauty products; but I assure you, once you get past the initial and painful hump, you're set.

Remember to always read labels as formulas can change. The most accurate information will always be directly on the product itself.

Ask the Manufacturer: If you're hooked on a beauty product and want to continue using it, but you're unsure if it contains gluten, ask the manufacturer. Sometimes you'll get a surprisingly clear answer; if you don't, it might just be the prompt you need to let it go. When in doubt, don't use the product. There are other fish in the sea and there is almost always a good alternative; it just takes a little time and effort to find your perfect match.

AT THE BEAUTY SHOP

I love to get mani-pedis, and most mani-pedis come complete with a wonderful lotion massage. Stop! Ask to look at the ingredients in those lotions they want to rub all over your hands and feet, and bring your own lotion, just in case. Many Bath and Body Works lotions (and even the brand's hand sanitizers) contain wheat germ.

CHAPTER 7
BEING WITHOUT YOU TAKES A LOT OF GETTING USED TO

"It's not just a matter of inadequate resolve, inconvenience, or breaking well-worn habits; it's about severing a relationship with something that gains hold of your psyche and emotions, not unlike the hold heroin has over the desperate addict."

– Dr. William Davis, author of Wheat Belly[54]

Breaking up with gluten is one thing, but living without the delicious protein is another. In fact, there are many times, especially in that first year, where I wanted to call upon gluten for a one-night stand.

To me, gluten was comfort food. I was emotionally connected to it. I couldn't imagine life without deep dish pizza, pasta, or sourdough bread bowls. I couldn't imagine a Thanksgiving without stuffing or buttery crescent rolls, a burger without a soft bun, a sandwich without bread, or mac and cheese without the mac. Like most Americans, I was undeniably addicted to gluten. I loved the way it tasted, and nothing excited me more than a big bowl of spaghetti (my mom will attest to this!).

I resisted, don't worry, but I know these cravings can be intense. In fact, Dr. William Davis, the author of *Wheat Belly*, says that for many people, wheat is an addictive substance, like an opiate, that can influence behavior and mood and even dominate thoughts. People who give up wheat go through distinct withdrawal symptoms that can make them nervous, foggy, tremulous, and desperately seeking another hit of wheat.[55] In fact, he says when people "divorce" themselves from wheat-containing products, 30 percent experience something that can only be called wheat withdrawal.[56] (Some experts contradict this, saying wheat withdrawal may only be found in about 10 percent of patients.[57]) He goes on to call wheat an "appetite stimulant" that makes you want more bread, cookies and cakes.[58] It's also why he notes that today, more than half of newly diagnosed celiac disease patients are classified as overweight or obese.[59] Perhaps an insatiable appetite for wheat is to blame?

In the days and months post-breakup with gluten, I was a mess. An absolute mess. I couldn't think straight, and I thought I was losing my mind. I was physically exhausted and overwhelmed from having to learn so much about my new "diet" so quickly. I couldn't stop thinking about food and life without gluten. I became irritable. Every little thing angered me from my kids leaving crumbs on the counter, to a frustrating encounter at a restaurant, and the sly comment from a well-meaning but uninformed friend.

For all intents and purposes, I was grumpy, both because I was physically going through gluten withdrawal and because I was mourning the loss of a once easy life. I used to eat anything I wanted without a care in the world. Now I had to pre-plan every meal, bring food along with me wherever I went (just in case), and have lengthy conversations about my diet with strangers in restaurants.

While I understood I was *just* giving up a food group, I began to have so much fear around food. I was nervous to eat anything and anxious about going out with friends. Even a wonderful dinner party at my best friend's house made me yearn to just stay home. On top of the fear of everyday eating, I also feared the future. What would become of me? Would I get cancer early and die? Will my nursing home have gluten-free options? What will life be like for me when I can't take care of myself?

While I was able to put it all in perspective, knowing that I could treat my "disease" with food and not some man-made pill or invasive surgical procedure, I also knew this special diet of mine would be a life-long prescription. And while I hated being *that person* who needed everyone to cater to her needs, the fact is this was my new reality, like it or not.

GETTING THROUGH WHEAT WITHDRAWAL

- **Hydrate Well:** Water will cool the inflammatory fire inside of you. Hunger and intense cravings can also be a sign of dehydration, so drink up.
- **Keep Healthy Snacks within Reach:** When hunger strikes, don't be stuck with nothing or you'll be tempted to eat gluten or junk food.
- **Stay Busy:** A busy person is less likely to think about food and nagging symptoms.
- **Eat Full Meals:** Eat full, well-balanced meals to keep you from feeling deprived. This is not a time to restrict calories or try to lose weight; rather this is a time to ease your body into a new and permanent way of eating. No meal skipping, either.
- **Load Up on Veggies:** Foods high in anti-oxidants will help boost your overall mental and physical health, allowing you to recover quickly from pesky withdrawal symptoms. We'll talk about more healing strategies in Part II.

A Hard Habit to Break

While I successfully made it through withdrawal symptoms and have never knowingly eaten gluten again after that last Subway sandwich, I realize that making the switch to the gluten-free way of life is easier said than done. I know so many people who struggle with it.

I have learned, however, that people with celiac disease have a greater adherence to the gluten-free diet than those with gluten sensitivity, even though gluten sensitivity can be just as serious. Ask someone who is intolerant to gluten how awful gluten makes them feel; you'll no doubt become more sympathetic to their plight.

I know several people with gluten disorders (including celiac disease) who have decided to continue to eat gluten despite the fact that it makes them sick. Obviously, everyone is different and has reasons for doing what they do. For me, I have many hopes and dreams about my future. I want to be here for a long time, and I don't want to be suffering through the last years of my life. If ditching gluten is what it takes to have the future I dream of, I'm all in.

Many people, however, are tempted to run back into gluten's not-so-loving arms for many reasons. They justify it by saying things like:

- "I'll have a piece of chocolate cake *just this once* because it's my birthday."
- "I really need a croissant to help me feel better after a really hard day."
- "I'm traveling next week, so I'm going to take a week off of the gluten-free diet."
- "A little gluten won't hurt me. It's not like I have celiac disease or anything *that* serious."
- "I have silent celiac, so I don't get any symptoms after eating gluten. That's why it's okay for me to have a little gluten."

Trust me, I've heard all of these reasons (err, excuses) for why people run back to their ex. It's not easy to watch, especially when you are trying to get people to take gluten free seriously.

The truth is that cheating on your gluten-free diet causes so much more damage than you may realize. I want to set the record straight that if you're following the gluten-free diet, you're on it. You're not gluten free when it's convenient or easy or when you feel like it. Whether you have celiac disease or gluten sensitivity, the only way you'll reap the long-term rewards of the gluten-free diet is by taking it seriously.

Let me be clear on why you should never, ever get back together with gluten:

You'll Undo All Your Progress: It only takes one small exposure to gluten to activate an immune system response (aka, attack). In other words, *just a little gluten* can and will hurt you.

You'll Feel Awful: Most of us feel awful after eating even a crumb of gluten. Some people will vomit. Others experience intense headaches, canker sores on their lips, urgent diarrhea, or itchy skin flareups. Why put yourself through that? Whatever symptoms you were trying to control by eating gluten free in the first place will come back – sometimes with a vengeance – when you start eating gluten again.

Your Risk for Other Autoimmune Diseases Increases: People who don't properly manage their autoimmune disease (celiac) are at a higher risk for accumulating additional autoimmune diseases. Even gluten sensitivity, which isn't formally classified as an autoimmune disease (yet), might be the trigger – or catalyst – that ripens your body for autoimmune disease. According to a study published in *Gastroenterology*,[60] people with a non-celiac wheat sensitivity (aka gluten sensitivity) have double the amount of elevated levels of antinuclear antibodies than the levels experienced in those with celiac disease. These are antibodies known to manifest themselves in autoimmune conditions like lupus, rheumatoid arthritis, Sjogren's syndrome, scleroderma, and polymyositis. In other words, if your exposure to gluten continues (e.g. by cheating on your gluten-free diet), you will likely progress further along the autoimmune spectrum, and your gluten sensitivity may eventually turn into a full-blown, irreversible autoimmune disease! Remember, celiac disease is just *one* manifestation of a sensitivity to wheat;[61] hundreds of other autoimmune conditions can be triggered by gluten or wheat.

Your Cancer Risk Increases: We all dread the C-word, and many of us have lost a loved one to cancer in our lifetime. Cancer can mean an early death sentence. For those who survive, it creates fear, stress, and trauma for years if not a lifetime. Persistent gut damage from eating gluten despite having celiac disease puts patients at serious risk of lymphoma, a type of blood cancer. In fact, a study published in the *Annals of Internal Medicine* found that people with celiac disease that incurred persistent intestinal damage had a higher risk of lymphoma than people whose intestines had healed. The best way to heal your intestinal lining is through strict adherence to a gluten-free diet.[62]

Another fascinating study performed by researchers at the Mayo Clinic found an increased prevalence and mortality rate in people with undiagnosed celiac disease. In the study, researchers tested frozen blood samples, drawn from 9,000 male Air Force recruits fifty years ago, for celiac disease. Researchers found that two percent of the recruits had undiagnosed celiac disease (double the currently accepted celiac disease rate), and that recruits with positive celiac disease markers were four times more likely to die over the next five decades, mainly from cancer, than the other recruits.[63]

Additional research continues to connect unmanaged celiac disease with a higher cancer risk. In an analysis of eight million residents of the United Kingdom, researchers observed 4,732 people with celiac disease along with five control subjects for each celiac participant. Over the three and a half years of observation, researchers found that those with celiac disease had a 30 percent greater likelihood of developing cancer, mostly gastrointestinal malignancies, and that one in 33 celiac participants developed cancer during the three-and-half-year observation period.[64]

(Interesting to note, this same study found that celiac patients had only one-third the risk for getting breast or lung cancer.)

Researchers in Sweden made similar observations about the connection between celiac disease and cancer, also showing a 30 percent increased risk for gastrointestinal cancers in patients with celiac disease, including malignant small intestinal lymphomas as well as cancer of the throat, esophagus, large intestine, liver, and pancreas.[65]

These findings suggest that intestinal healing should be the ultimate goal for patients with celiac disease in order to stave off cancer. The delicate intestinal lining cannot heal if you repeatedly eat gluten, even if only on occasion.

You'll Die Early: Death is inevitable, and being diagnosed with an autoimmune condition makes you take your mortality more seriously. Despite widespread awareness of celiac disease and greater access to gluten-free food, the risk of premature death from cardiovascular disease, cancer and respiratory disease is 21 percent higher in people with celiac disease than the general population.[66] The reasons you are following the gluten-free diet are to reclaim your health, avoid being one of those chronically ill people who can't enjoy life, and, of course, deter early death.

A study published in the *Lancet* followed celiac patients for more than 20 years and recorded their eating patterns. Patients who ate gluten once per month, even if they didn't feel bad after eating gluten, incurred a six-fold increase in the relative risk of death.[67] In other words, researchers found that patients with poor compliance to the gluten-free diet were at the highest risk for early death, and that "strict" dietary treatment decreases mortality in celiac patients.

In another study published in *The Journal of the American Medical Association*, researchers set out to examine the mortality rates in people with celiac disease compared to those with *just* inflamed intestines. They examined approximately 46,000 people with celiac disease and about 13,000 subjects with gluten sensitivity and intestinal inflammation (they had neither positive bloodwork for celiac disease nor worn-down microvilli).

Researchers found that subjects with celiac disease had a 39 percent increased risk of early mortality while those with inflammation from gluten sensitivity had a 72 percent increased risk of early mortality.[6869] In other words, people with gluten sensitivity had a higher likelihood of dying early than those with full-blown celiac disease. Why is that?

I can't say for sure why people with inflammation have a higher early mortality rate than those with full-blown celiac. However, I suspect that people with gluten sensitivity may not fully manage their disorder through strict adherence to the gluten-free diet, whereas people with celiac disease take their disorder more seriously. Regardless, this study offers clear evidence that whether you have celiac disease or gluten sensitivity, eating *just a little* gluten has serious, life-threatening consequences.

No One Will Take You Seriously: On top of it all, if you continually cheat on your gluten-free diet, how will anyone take you seriously if you don't even take yourself seriously? Your cavalier attitude towards having *just* one sip of beer at a restaurant conditions other people to believe this gluten thing is a bunch of baloney. Either you're gluten free or you're not. You can't have it both ways.

One of my least favorite comments is when people say to me, "I tried eating gluten free, and it didn't work for me." I know these people rarely give gluten free a fair shake, and it doesn't take a rocket scientist to know that most "diets" don't work when they're approached as a diet vs. lifestyle change. The "diet" also doesn't work if you continue to hook up with gluten.

I also hear people say, "I used to be gluten free, but I feel better so I can eat gluten again." The reason you feel better is because you avoided gluten and your body healed. Now that you're back with your ex, it has the ability to hurt you all over again. There's no need to return to an abusive relationship if you're feeling just fine on your own.

This reminds me of a story I read on the NPR website about the early discovery of celiac disease. Doctors believed that a diet that forbade starches and included a daily banana, along with milk, cottage cheese, meat, and vegetables, would "cure" celiac disease. In the early 1920s, parents would look to Dr. Sidney Haas in California to treat their babies suffering from this little-known nutritional disorder. Dr. Haas would care for these babies for six months, feeding them the "banana" diet.

After six months, Dr. Haas would declare the babies "cured" and return them to their families. We know now that the bananas did not "cure" the babies; it was the omission of gluten in their diets that was responsible for their intestinal healing. Once they went back on a gluten-y diet, their symptoms returned.

One of those banana babies, Lindy Redmond, told NPR, "All my life I have told doctors I had celiac disease as a child and that I grew out of it. And all my life I have eaten wheat." It was only when she was 66 years old that her doctors tested her again for celiac disease and found intestinal damage. She told NPR that she wondered if unmanaged celiac disease was connected to her miscarriages, frequent colds, and endless constipation.[70]

The point of this story is to reiterate that celiac disease is not curable, and just because you feel better doesn't mean you're "cured." The truth is that only lifelong adherence to the gluten-free diet will keep intestinal damage at bay. Too often patients suffering from gluten disorders are mistakenly told that they are cured and can once again eat gluten. When you go back to eating gluten, the vicious cycle of damage begins anew.

WE ARE NEVER, EVER, GETTING BACK TOGETHER

Once you break it off with gluten, there's no going back. It's over. Kaput. It's time to make this breakup official. It's time to update your relationship status on Facebook.

If you go back to gluten, you might find some weird things happening, making you realize once and for all that gluten is no good for you. While there is no research dedicated to exploring gluten reexposure, anecdotally people have told me that after reintroducing gluten, their symptoms came back with a vengeance. They don't just experience bloating; they experience intense and painful bloating. They suddenly find themselves experiencing joint pain or new symptoms like itchy skin or migraines. They report their symptoms last longer and are more pronounced than they were prior to the split. Some people report feeling like they've been poisoned.

Consider yourself warned.

Handling Accidental Gluten Exposure

While it doesn't happen often, I have, on occasion, been exposed to gluten without knowing it. It's usually after eating at a friend's house, a restaurant, or eating something new. I feel an urgent need to use the bathroom, I experience intense bloating and stomach pangs, and I typically suffer from a few bouts of diarrhea until my body fully purges the offending protein from my system.

That said, because I have put in the hard work to heal my gut, an accidental gluten exposure typically passes quickly for me. Within an hour or two, I feel better and can function again. I know everyone is different, and an accidental exposure can set some people back more than others. You might experience different symptoms, and the severity of those symptoms can depend on whether you ate something that came in cross-contact with gluten, or you unknowingly ate an entire gluten-full pizza. Work hard at keeping your gut healthy and building your immune system so that you are able to more quickly bounce back from an accidental gluten exposure. (I'll talk more about how to heal your gut and build immunity in Part II.)

If you've been accidentally glutened, try some of these home remedies to ease your symptoms and to recover more quickly. Remember, this too shall pass, literally!

Hydrate Like Crazy: Flush the gluten out of your system and replenish any water lost from vomiting and/or diarrhea. Lemon water is very alkalizing and can help you more quickly restore your body's natural pH balance.

Rest: Stay close to home when you've been glutened, and rest up. Rest will help your digestive system relax and restore. And if you're experiencing any sort of intestinal distress, staying close to your own bathroom is a must.

Rest Your Digestive System: Allow your digestive system time to rest and recover by fasting for a few hours or eating easy-to-digest foods like broths, rice, bananas, gluten-free crackers, and tea (with lemon and/or ginger) to help settle your stomach. Avoid overeating. See Chapter 11 for additional strategies for resting your digestive system.

Add Beneficial Bacteria to Your Gut: In Chapter 10, I will talk about the benefits of probiotics. In times of accidental gluten exposure, you may want to consider doubling up on your probiotic dosage, taking one dose in the AM and the second dose in the PM in order to give your gut an extra boost of beneficial bacteria in this time of crisis. Please consult your doctor for dosage recommendations.

Take Activated Charcoal: Activated charcoal is typically used to treat poisonings or drug overdoses. Toxins bind to the charcoal, which helps the body rid itself of these unwanted substances. This claim, however, has not been scientifically validated.

Take a Digestive Enzyme: Our bodies produce a plethora of digestive enzymes naturally. These enzymes help break down and improve the absorption of food. Today, however, you can purchase supplements to increase the number of digestive enzymes in your body and aid in the breakdown of food. There are many digestive enzymes available, but one that many people have recommended to me is called GlutenEase™, which is marketed as a digestive supplement to be taken only during accidental gluten exposure. GlutenEase is said to assist in the breakdown of gluten and gliadin proteins. (I do not endorse GlutenEase nor have I tried it.)

Please note that the overuse of digestive enzymes may "teach" your body's naturally enzyme-producing cells to stop producing these enzymes, tricking your body into thinking it already has enough of them. Therefore, digestive enzymes should be used to augment, not replace, the body's natural digestive enzymes. Use digestive enzymes only in times of need, such as an accidental gluten exposure.

IT TAKES GUTS: SHANNON FORD'S IMPROVED RELATIONSHIP WITH FOOD

Shannon Ford is a consummate star in the pageant world, having been crowned Mrs. United States (2011), Mrs. Florida America (2019), and third runner-up Mrs. America (2019). She also is a former Miami Dolphins cheerleader and a celiac disease warrior.

Like many people, Ford was diagnosed with the autoimmune disorder as an adult, at the age of 31. It all started in 2009 when Ford began to suffer from chronic fatigue. Her doctor diagnosed her with hypothyroidism. Despite taking medication for her thyroid condition, her fatigue lingered.

On top of experiencing chronic fatigue, Ford was under a lot of stress at work. As a human resources manager, she recalls a difficult, stress-inducing journey across the U.S. where she was charged with laying off dozens of workers. She crashed when she finally arrived at home. She says she usually rests for a few days and is back in business, but this time was different. Ford could barely get out of bed.

Ford's fatigue persisted for 10 months with no answers from her doctors. Everything changed, however, when she saw an interview on TV with talk-show host, Elisabeth Hasselbeck. Hasselbeck, who at the time was promoting her gluten-free diet book, described having intense fatigue and bloating that caused her to look pregnant after she ate. She notes these were all symptoms of undiagnosed and unmanaged celiac disease.

Ford adds that her fiancé (now husband) said to her as they watched the interview, "That's it; that's what you have." The couple had always joked that Ford looked like she was carrying a 'baby pizza' or 'pasta baby' after eating carbs.

Ford returned to her doctor and asked to be tested for celiac disease. A few days later, she received the answer she'd been searching for. She had celiac disease. It was official.

Like many people who struggle with their health for years, Ford found her diagnosis a relief.

"I was never sad about it. My attitude was, 'If you're going to have a disease, this is a good one to have.' It had been close to a year of being told nothing was wrong with me and not feeling well. To finally have an answer made me happy, and losing gluten, to me, was an easy fix," she admits.

The other benefit to having celiac disease, adds Ford, is that it taught her to have a better relationship with food.

"You have this weird relationship with food in the pageant world. While I was thin, I wasn't necessarily healthy. This is why celiac disease has been a blessing in disguise. I ate to not be fat, things like Lean Cuisine meals and Nutrisystem protein shakes, but eliminating gluten made me focus on eating whole foods and realize that food is fuel. I am definitely healthier. Celiac changed my relationship with food for the better," she says.

Almost two years after diagnosis, Ford went on to be crowned Mrs. United States and she made celiac disease her platform.

"Advisors told me I would never win with celiac disease as my platform because it wasn't 'big enough,' but I didn't care because I wanted to help people, make celiac disease mainstream, and bring awareness to an illness that a lot of people suffer from but don't know about," she insists, adding that at the time she was crowned Mrs. United States, there weren't even gluten-free labeling regulations in place.

Today, Ford tells others to surround themselves with a good support system, and always demand better of restaurants and others. She adds, "It didn't take me long to learn that no one is going to care about my health more than me."

CHAPTER 8
THE EMOTIONAL BURDEN OF
THE GLUTEN-FREE DIET

"Our painful experiences aren't a liability – they're a gift. They give us perspective and meaning, an opportunity to find our unique purpose and our strength."

– Dr. Edith Eger

Breaking up with gluten comes with a roller coaster of emotions, which will be different for everyone. People who have been struggling with their health for a long time with no answers will often say they experienced intense feelings of relief when they were diagnosed. They say they finally understood what was happening to their bodies and what they could do about it.

Actress Casey Wilson shared her story with the *New York Times*, saying that when she finally found out her two-year-old son had celiac disease, she experienced "unimaginable relief." Within months, she says her son went from "melancholy" and "depressed" to "thriving" and "bursting with life."[71]

While most people are relieved to finally have a diagnosis, especially those who have been ill for so long without explanation, many people will then collide with feelings of shock, grief, anger, resentment, and fear as they begin to dive into the nitty-gritty daily realities involved with living a medically necessary gluten-free life.

One topic I have talked about on my blog is the significant emotional burden of having a gluten disorder and following a gluten-free diet. This emotional burden can hit you at any time.

As I'm writing this, almost eight years into my gluten-free journey, I realize that I am not immune to this emotional burden. In fact, just recently I was attending a special event for 300 people in my community. I requested a gluten-free meal ahead of time and confirmed the day prior with the event coordinator that the gluten-free meal was still a go. Yet, when I arrived at my table to eat, it turned out that getting a gluten-free meal would still be a challenge despite my best efforts.

Throughout the meal, I watched those around me enjoy appetizers. None for me. I watched my friends enjoy bread and special dips. None for me. Then, when the main course came, I had to wait until everyone was served before the caterer presented me with my "safe" meal. I felt humiliated and uncomfortable sitting at the table while those around me feasted. Everyone at my table was on to their third course while I was waiting for my first. Trust me, I wasn't starving, and I didn't expect people to cater to me. But I had requested the meal, and the caterer had said "no problem." I was anticipating being able to eat alongside everyone else. This whole incident made me feel isolated and frustrated. I found myself holding back tears as I tried to keep myself composed despite the emotional burden.

BETRAYED BY A PROMISING TRIP

In 2019 I went on the trip of a lifetime to Israel, a place I have visited in the past and where I always dream of going back. I went with a women's tour group and had a full itinerary of travels and lectures. The trip was all-inclusive, meaning the vast majority of meals would be included and part of the tour. Of course, before I agreed to go on the trip I spoke with my city leader and the leader of the entire trip. They both assured me that providing me with safe, gluten-free meals would be "no problem."

Unfortunately, however, getting a gluten-free meal turned out to be a major problem. The chef who was catering food for our tour group was paralyzed with fear when it came to preparing food for me. The staff was ill-prepared to host me despite my earlier inquiries and assurance.

On top of that, I did not want to leave the tour group. I would have missed out on all the lectures that happened during meal time. The benefit of going through a tour group is that the tour leaders are supposed to take care of those all-inclusive details for you.

Of course, Israel has all sorts of gluten-free food. This is a nation known for its delicious and healthy Mediterranean fare. However, I was at the whim of my tour group. I was stuck. While my friends feasted on bread and gourmet meals, I nibbled on lettuce, carrots and the few packaged food items I brought with me (aka, my emergency stash). I did not get warm meals, nor beautiful foods to eat like everyone else on my tour group. I simply ate to survive.

By day three I was fed up, quite literally. I was sick of advocating for myself and feeling hungry. I had been holding back tears, but as an emotional person, eventually the tears flowed like Niagara Falls. It happened while we were "eating" at a restaurant. My tour group leader told me the restaurant would have a "safe" meal for me, finally. As I watched my group dine on several courses of beautiful foods provided by the restaurant staff, I patiently waited for the "safe" meal I was assured would be coming for me.

About midway through dinner, my "safe" meal arrived. It was a sad, unseasoned, and overcooked chicken breast over white bean sprouts. I couldn't believe no one in this beautiful country could create a warm, safe, nourishing meal for me. After the meal, everyone was having a great time, but I was busy holding back tears. Food is meant to bring joy, but I felt only sad and defeated. I left the restaurant in tears while my friends stayed and danced. Their bellies were full, their bodies well-nourished.

Even as I write this, there is a lump in my throat. It may seem trivial to most people – perhaps a "first world problem" as some would say – but to me, I felt like a burden, a social pariah; on top of it all, my emotions were getting the best of me. I might have been a little hangry, too. I had not eaten properly for three days, and I was exhausted having to explain myself over and over again.

I'm usually tougher than that. However, despite my educating, pleading, and advocating, this "no-food-for-Jenny" routine continued for the rest of my trip. I was promised a meal and sorely disappointed by the sad plate of food placed before me. Again, I didn't starve, and I had bars and fruit with me, and I stopped at a few places to pick up food for myself along the way, but I'd much rather receive a beautiful, warm meal like everyone else.

I shared my humbling story on Instagram only to find that so many others have experienced similar situations. I learned that everyone's emotions are high when it happens to them. That is when I realized I am not alone in carrying the emotional burden that comes with having celiac disease and eating gluten free.

FEAR AND ANXIETY

Some people, including myself at times, feel paralyzed by their gluten-free diet. They refuse to travel, eat at restaurants, or attend business functions that involve food for fear of being "poisoned" by gluten. No one wants to be accidentally glutened and find themselves a few hours later laid up on the couch or stuck on the toilet. Many people who have been severely glutened wind up with flu-like symptoms. A good friend of mine actually ended up in the ER, feeling sick to her stomach and severely dehydrated, after eating gluten. She ate a piece of regular pizza before the waiter realized she had given her the wrong pizza!

Besides the fear of accidentally eating gluten, many fear the potential of having to face an awkward social interaction. I often wonder, "What will my friends think of me after they see how I interrogate the waiter and sound like such a diva when I place my order?" This fear of confrontation and having to look "different" from everyone else is sometimes more paralyzing to me than the fear of getting glutened!

The truth is, we all get to choose how we respond when fear takes hold. I learned from Dr. Edith Eger, in her book, *The Choice*, that in difficult situations, we can choose to be miserable, or we can choose to be hopeful. We can choose to be depressed, or we can choose to be happy.[72] The choice is ours and this is why I don't let my fear and anxiety rule my life. This is why, despite knowing the risk of having no food available to me, I still choose to travel and eat out. I choose to live my life (with a few adjustments, of course).

ISOLATION AND SADNESS

Following a gluten-free diet can also make you feel isolated. A few years ago I was walking by a bakery with a group of friends. They decided to go in and buy treats as the bakery's wonderful scents were wafting in the air, enticing each passerby. My friends purchased boxes of pastries while I waited outside and felt sorry for myself.

I could see the excitement in their eyes when they were shopping, and they were excited to share their "finds" with me and one another. I had to pretend to be excited by their purchases. I didn't want to be a Debbie Downer nor have them feel guilty for indulging in something perfectly normal.

In a survey mailed to patients with celiac disease, gastroesophageal reflux disease (GERD), irritable bowel syndrome, inflammatory bowel disease, hypertension (HTN), diabetes mellitus (DM), congestive heart failure, and end-stage renal disease (ESRD) on dialysis, researchers set out to understand the burden of treatment for each disorder. The study included 341 celiac participants and 368 non-celiac participants. Celiac disease participants reported a much higher treatment burden than those with GERD or HTN and comparable to those with ESRD. However, interestingly enough, celiac disease participants had the most excellent overall health status in comparison to individuals with the other chronic medical conditions surveyed. (Pretty good silver lining, right?) Researchers concluded that the significant burden faced by patients of celiac disease makes a strong case for the need for additional treatment options and interventions.[73]

Depression rates are also higher for those who follow a gluten-free diet than the general population.[74] Researchers found that even among individuals managing their illness "very well," participants still report higher rates of stress and depression and a range of issues including body dissatisfaction (weight and shape) when compared to the general population.[75] I can attest to these feelings. I manage my illness "very well," and am mentally strong; but there are times when emotions overcome me, and I can't help but feel sad and isolated on this journey.

Dr. Eger says that isolation is a form of imprisonment, whereas accepting what is and understanding that your suffering has meaning, is freedom.[76] Over the years, I have gone from "why me?" to "why not me?" This change in perspective has helped me discover the meaning of celiac disease in my life.

STRESSFUL RELATIONSHIPS

The emotional burden of the gluten-free diet doesn't just impact the person with the disorder; it can also adversely impact those who care for a person on the diet. A study from Columbia University found that caregivers experience high levels of stress, anxiety and emotional burden when it came to caring for someone with celiac disease, particularly a patient with severe symptoms. Interestingly, the researchers found that "burden scores" experienced by caregivers of celiac disease patients to be "remarkably similar" to the reported burden scores of those caring for patients of other chronic diseases including terminal cancer. The researchers note that while this study was not designed to compare the burden among disease processes, it does highlight that caring for someone with celiac disease takes a fair amount of "understanding, acceptance and support from loved ones."[77]

I recently watched my friend deal with the emotional burden of raising a child with celiac disease, particularly in the early months. My friend's daughter (we'll call her Kate) goes to a private sleepaway camp every year. Unfortunately, Kate was diagnosed with celiac disease about four months before the start of camp.

When my friend called the camp to request accommodations for Kate, the camp told her to take her business elsewhere. They said they were a private camp and simply could not accommodate one child with special gluten-free food when they're trying to feed 500 children simultaneously. Apparently the camp has the right to do this. My friend said Kate was devastated. All her friends go to this camp, and this seemingly "normal" experience has been ripped from her. Talk about an emotional burden you never want your 13-year-old daughter to have to face. The emotions are raw, and the struggle is real.

Dating is another emotional burden that can impact your mental state. If you're dating while following a gluten-free diet, your special diet usually comes up prior to the first date because you'll have to explain that you can eat only at certain restaurants. If it doesn't come up before the date, it will certainly come up on the date as you explain your diet – in front of your date – to a potentially doubting waiter. What other disease would you have to explain to someone on a first date? A 2018 survey found that more than 40 percent of people say they would be "reluctant" to date someone who avoids gluten because they perceive gluten-free eaters as "high maintenance."[78] The emotional burden of the gluten-free diet can become compounded if your date loves to eat gluten. Your date may have downed a beer or two, along with his or her burger (with bun). Have fun explaining why your date doesn't get a goodnight kiss!

DISCOVERING MEANING

While emotions run high and all of us feel the burden of the gluten-free diet at some point, I urge you to continue to advocate for what you need and for what is right. My friend went to Israel with the same tour group one year later. She, too, is serious about eating gluten free. She told me there were "plenty" of gluten-free options provided just for her, and that food was a "non-issue."

It struck me, at that moment, that my suffering had meaning. I had paved the way for her and perhaps others who need special accommodations during their travels. My frustrations and tears had not been in vain. There is a glimmer of light even in the darkest of situations.

IT TAKES GUTS: PATRICK STAROPOLI'S COURSE CORRECTION

Patrick Staropoli has a lot going for him. He is a graduate of Harvard University and University of Miami Medical Center, and is working towards completing his residency in ophthalmology.

However, Staropoli may be best known as a professional stock car racer, a once-in-a-lifetime dream opportunity he earned after winning the 2013 PEAK® Stock Car Dream Challenge, a reality-TV competition search for the best amateur racer. After winning the competition, Staropoli had the opportunity to compete on the NASCAR circuit and at legendary race tracks such as Daytona and Bristol, and he continues to compete to this day as time and resources permit.

Staropoli's rise to success has not always been a smooth ride. In fact, a health scare in 2010, when Staropoli was a sophomore in college, forever altered the course of his life.

Staropoli discovered a strange ulcer in his throat. An endoscopy examination revealed good and bad news. The good news was that the ulcer had almost completely healed. The bad news was that Staropoli's intestines were damaged in a way consistent with celiac disease. A biopsy confirmed his doctor's suspicions, and Staropoli was officially diagnosed with celiac disease.

Staropoli says he was in a state of "shock" when his doctor told him the news. He went in for one disorder and came out with another. Like 20 percent of celiac patients, Staropoli was asymptomatic. He had never experienced GI symptoms congruent with celiac disease, and no one in his family had the disorder at that time. (His father and grandmother were later diagnosed with celiac disease.)

"At first I never knew if something I ate had been cross-contaminated with gluten or if there was a hidden [gluten] ingredient causing damage to my intestines. Being asymptomatic made it hard for me to find the motivation to change my whole lifestyle – especially during college when most students are surviving on ramen noodles and pizza," he says.

Despite being asymptomatic, Staropoli says he was determined to figure out the gluten-free diet, and was ready to go the extra mile to eat in a way that worked best for his body.

Over the years, he says he began to experience celiac-related GI symptoms, and now notices that even a little gluten makes him feel very ill. He can't help but wonder if he's become sensitized to gluten or if it's just the natural progression of the disease.

Today, Staropoli says he is a pro at living the gluten-free lifestyle. He is comfortable eating at home and at restaurants, although he admits that the social aspects of the disease are a constant struggle.

"You get the feeling you are the limiting factor when picking a dinner spot or planning an event. It's awkward when you have to order Uber Eats at a wedding because the caterer didn't make anything gluten free," he laments.

The good news, he says, is there are many more gluten-free options at restaurants and stores today than when he was first diagnosed, and living the gluten-free lifestyle is getting easier each day, albeit never easy.

He also says celiac disease has not changed his race prep one bit, apart from the fact that he has converted his pit crew to eating gluten free.

"On race days I stick to yogurt and hard-boiled eggs for breakfast, roll up cold cuts and cheese for lunch, and constantly hydrate throughout the day. Racetrack food is an interesting culinary experience that's probably similar to eating street food when you travel internationally. It's tempting, but I definitely stay away from that now," he says.

Staropoli advises others diagnosed with celiac disease to take it in stride and keep things in perspective.

"I remember thinking when I was first diagnosed that there are much worse things I could have been diagnosed with and that this is something I can manage. With the popularization of the diet, it has become much easier to learn and follow. It has not held me back in any way from the goals I have set for myself in school, on the racetrack, or even now working in the hospital," he says.

On the bright side, his favorite meal of steak, potatoes, and vegetables has always been gluten free, and he is willing to make a pit stop anywhere in search of the perfect gluten-free black-and-white cookie.

PART II

THE HEALING

CHAPTER 9
I'M JUST NOT THAT INTO YOU

"A person who has health has a thousand dreams. A person who does not, has just one. And, it's to feel better. When you can give someone their health back, they can go after all of their dreams."

– Dr. Izabella Wentz

I thought by breaking things off with gluten my life would instantly be better. I thought my painful bloating would completely disappear, and that I'd be saying so long to embarrassing gas for good. How wrong I was!

Following a gluten-free diet isn't the cure-all it's made out to be, and while most people report feeling better after ditching gluten, their symptoms are not fully a thing of the past, and oftentimes their symptoms reemerge, often overtime, despite eating gluten free. Why is healing so difficult?

For starters, the damage caused by gluten has been brewing inside someone for years, and therefore the wounds are deep. It takes an average of four years for a symptomatic person with celiac disease to be diagnosed[79] (some studies report up to 11 years![80]), meaning the damage is pervasive. A gluten disorder leaves your gut in shambles, your body in a chronic state of nutrient-deprivation, and often is the catalyst for a slew of other ailments. Recurring, insidious damage to your body formed over years of eating gluten can take years – and more than *only* eating gluten free – to eradicate.

Furthermore, complete gut healing isn't an easy feat for most patients of celiac disease. A study of 465 celiac disease patients found that even though most reported feeling better after their initial split with gluten, only eight percent had normal tissue while most continued to show underlying, excessive inflammation in their intestines. Researchers concluded that "complete normalization" of the tissue surrounding the small intestine was "exceptionally rare" in adult celiac patients despite adherence to the gluten-free diet, symptom disappearance, and a negative blood test.[81] This study demonstrates just how difficult it is to achieve full remission by eating *only* gluten-free food, and perhaps suggests there is more that patients need to do to completely heal. It also demonstrates that feeling better doesn't always equate to complete intestinal healing.

Another reason full healing is difficult for people with gluten disorders is the fact that gluten is everywhere and difficult to avoid. In fact, strict adherence to the gluten-free diet is near impossible if you eat out or consume any packaged foods. Even if someone is able to ignore all temptations of gluten, it still hides in our food and can be served to us by well-meaning friends and restaurants who say they understand gluten free but don't. Even a little gluten crumb here and there will continue to damage your body and impair complete healing.

Finally, I believe complete healing from a gluten disorder is hard because maybe, just maybe, conventional wisdom is wrong. Doctors and researchers tell people with gluten disorders to eat gluten free and eventually they will feel better. This may be true for some people, but if I've learned anything over my eight-year battle with celiac disease, and my hundreds of conversations with others suffering from gluten disorders, it's that there is no one-size-fits-all approach to healing from celiac disease. Eating gluten free *may* completely heal one person, but what I have found personally, and in so many conversations with people in the gluten-free community, is that most people feel only marginally better after splitting with gluten, or they feel better at first, then relapse and begin to question the gluten-free diet and whether it's worth it after all.

I've personally come to the conclusion that the gluten-free diet isn't a cure-all. Sure, gluten has got to go and it's the reason you're in this mess in the first place, but it's not the *only* change you need to make to restore your health. Gluten has damaged your body for years in a deep, permeating way, and it *may* take more than eating gluten-free donuts to fix your broken body.

NURTURE THY WOUNDS

Imagine you've been stabbed in the gut with a knife. If you simply remove the knife, are you cured of that knife wound? No! The truth is, you must nurture the wound left behind if you want to survive. If you don't, you will surely bleed to death or suffer from a painful and life-threatening infection. Now replace the knife in this analogy with gluten. You can remove gluten from your diet, but what are you doing to address the wound left behind?

I believe there is much more to healing your body after a celiac disease or gluten sensitivity diagnosis than simply removing the pesky protein.

Coming to this realization prompted me to experiment with various healing techniques and made me more determined than ever to fix my broken body, put my symptoms in remission, and restore my health. I wasn't sure *how* I was going to do this, but at least I was now asking the right questions. I no longer needed to know how to eat gluten free, but now I needed to know how to eat in a way that healed my body and was good for me.

WHAT DOCTORS DON'T KNOW MIGHT HURT YOU

You must become more knowledgeable than your doctor(s) when it comes to "treating" your gluten disorder. The truth is that doctors didn't learn everything there is to know about gluten sensitivities and celiac disease in medical school. Your physician may have heard a grumbling or two about gluten, but chances are it was far from the focus of his or her training. On top of that, doctors receive very little, if any, nutrition training. U.S. medical schools offer only 19.6 hours of nutrition courses during the average four-year program.[82] Given the fact that most Americans, at some time in their life, have asked their doctor for advice about their diet, this statistic is disturbing.

On top of having little nutrition training, doctors have limited time to spend with patients. Most visits to the doctor average 22 minutes, leaving little time for a discussion about chronic illness and unexplained symptoms, much less how to eat gluten free.[83] It's no wonder that the average time from symptoms to a formal diagnosis of celiac disease is four or more years!

I tell you this not to insult doctors. In fact, doctors play an important role in helping us research and understand gluten disorders. I'm simply telling you that the system today isn't set up for doctors to help patients suffering from chronic illnesses. Many of the doctors we turn to for help have never learned, in earnest, about the role of food in promoting good health. Medical schools spend a disproportionate amount of time teaching budding doctors about pharmaceuticals than they do about nutrition, leaving doctors in the lurch about how food affects every cell, organ, and tissue in our bodies. If nutrition was the centerpiece of medical wisdom, doctors would learn that food is either causing inflammation or promoting health. And they'd learn that throwing a bunch of pills at something won't work if someone is eating all the wrong foods.

I hope the information in the following pages inspires you to take matters into your own hands. To trust your gut. To use food as your medicine. To be your best advocate. To become more knowledgeable than your doctor. And to repair your body using food.

Your Body Is Programmed to Heal

Healing is possible, and you must never lose hope that your body can heal from the deep damage caused by your ex. Your body is an incredible vessel. It's programmed to heal – even restore – itself if given the chance.

Think about a time when you cut your finger. In just a few days, you hardly notice something went awry. Your finger is back to normal. Your body did that. Incredible, right? Your body is programmed to heal itself. But let's say you continue to use and reinjure that cut finger over and over again. The injury will turn into something much worse and it cannot fully heal until you stop reinjuring it.

Now apply this logic to your broken digestive system. Gluten has impaired your digestive system for a long time, and every time you eat gluten, you reinjure your gut over and over again. Your damaged gut cannot heal, restore, or function properly if you continue to eat gluten or assault it with other damaging foods, which I'll talk about more in this section.

Furthermore, it's important to note that there are no simple, quick, or cheap fixes to healing your body. There are no magical pills, potions, or procedures. There's just you, the food on your plate, and your own personal commitment to turning your health around. There's no short-cut to being healthy. You have to put in the hard work to create health in your life; no one is going to do it for you.

Healing vs. Curing

Please note that healing and curing are two different things. You cannot be cured of a gluten disorder. For those who have celiac disease or gluten sensitivity, the disorders will always require proper attention and management. However, symptoms can go away, and that starts with, as Dr. O'Bryan often says, the food at the end of your fork.

While you cannot be cured of a gluten disorder, you can heal from one, both physically and emotionally. You can put your symptoms into remission, and live a healthy, symptom-free, and meaningful life if you properly manage your disorder.

Dr. Kelly Turner, the author of the *New York Times* bestselling book *Radical Remission: Surviving Cancer Against All Odds*, helped me understand the difference between healing and curing in such a meaningful and eloquent way: "Curing means getting rid of a disease, while healing means becoming whole. Curing is *sometimes* possible, while healing is *always* possible. Healing simply means bringing more purpose, happiness, and healthy behaviors into your life."[84]

I believe you have the power to heal – and bring more meaning to your newfound life without gluten, and I'm excited to share how to do that. Remember, as you read the following healing strategies, that everyone heals differently, and no one heals in a straight line. You are a unique bio-individual, and I encourage you to experiment with different strategies until you figure out what works best for you. As always, consult your health care team before making any changes to your diet, taking any supplements, or changing medications.

CHAPTER 10
A GUT-WRENCHING BREAKUP

"The intuitive mind is a sacred gift and the rational mind is a faithful servant. We have created a society that honors the servant and has forgotten the gift."

– Albert Einstein

Think about a time when you were really nervous to do something. Maybe you had to speak or perform in front of a large audience, participate in a nerve-wracking interview, or were under a lot of pressure to get a good grade or nail a client presentation. Before your "performance," you felt butterflies in your stomach, and all the pent-up, nervous energy and excitement was brewing inside your gut.

Your gut often feels things before the rest of your body because your gut is lined with some 100 million neurons, more neurons than found in either your spinal cord or peripheral nervous system.[85] Your gut is, for all intents and purposes, your second brain.

Not only is your gut your second brain, but one could argue that it's the most important organ in your body. Your gut is literally responsible for feeding all your other organs. Without proper nutrient distribution, how will you fuel your hardworking brain and body?

Unfortunately, when a gluten disorder has taken hold of your body, your gut is damaged. However, just because you removed the offending protein doesn't mean your job of mending your broken gut is done. In fact, you have a long road to recovery ahead of you. And it all starts inside your second brain.

FEED YOUR GUT WELL

The community of bacteria, yeast, and viruses that live in your gut is collectively known as the microbiome. Only in the last few decades has the microbiome begun to be recognized as a key factor in your whole-body health. Your microbiome can weigh up to five pounds (your brain weighs half that!), and each living organism in your gut is made up of its own cells and genes. In fact, you have 150 times more genes in your gut alone, and your gut harbors more than a thousand different bacteria species. It's no wonder that 70-85 percent of the immune system resides inside the gut![86]

Your microbiome is controlled by your genetics, your environment, and the foods you eat. This is why it's essential to nurture your gut with foods that *promote* health rather than take away from it. In fact, a poorly fed microbiome crammed with gluten and other inflammatory foods is notoriously filled with bad bacteria and unwanted yeast, and it's ripe for nasty bugs and viruses to survive and grow.

It's important to note that your genes do not cause disease; rather, they simply reveal where you have a genetic predisposition or vulnerability toward a disease. Just because you carry the gene for celiac disease doesn't mean you'll *get* celiac disease. Other factors must occur, such as continuous consumption of gluten and intestinal permeability. For example, if you carry one of the celiac disease genes but don't eat any gluten, your celiac genes will not "turn on" and your blood test will come back negative for celiac disease each and every time. To quote Dr. Perlmutter, the author of *Grain Brain*, "Food is a powerful epigenetic modulator – meaning it can change our DNA for better or worse."[87]

This means that what you put on your plate directly influences the expression of your genes.

FEED YOUR BODY ANTI-INFLAMMATORY FOODS

Gluten is like a weapon of mass destruction to your gut. It not only causes inflammation in all who eat it, but the worst collateral damage is found in those with celiac disease or gluten sensitivity. I cannot emphasize enough that there is more to healing your body than simply splitting with gluten. In fact, what you *remove* from your diet is just as important as what you *put back into it.* If you're replacing wheat bread with gluten-free bread, swapping pizza for gluten-free pizza, and eating gluten-free pasta in lieu of wheat pasta, you're hardly feeding your gut right. This is why putting good stuff back in is an essential step to accelerate the healing of your gut.

Eating plenty of anti-inflammatory foods each and every day will aid in healing your body from the inside out. Your nutrient bank has been depleted from years of gluten consumption and bad eating habits, and now, more than ever, it needs nutrient-dense foods that serve to replenish, restore, and heal your gut.

Below are some of the many anti-inflammatory foods that will refuel your gut – and whole body:

Vegetables: Enjoy any and all vegetables, raw, cooked, steamed, blended or juiced. Enjoy them however you like them. You can't go wrong. Green, leafy vegetables are among the most nutrient-dense produce in the world, so load up on kale, spinach, collard greens and Swiss chard. All vegetables will promote health in your body, so eat the rainbow and enjoy asparagus, bell peppers, zucchini, squash, tomatoes, cucumbers, celery, carrots and more.

Fruits: Fruits are nature's perfectly packaged dessert. Enjoy fruit when you crave a little sweetness. Unlike pure sugar, which depletes your nutrient reserves during digestion, a piece of fruit comes with its own set of nutrients and fiber to help you properly digest the fruit while keeping your nutrient bank full.

A good rule of thumb is to fill half of your plate with vegetables and fruits so you load up on these *good for you* foods and leave less room for other foods that don't build your nutrient reserves. The other half of your plate should be filled with lean proteins and gluten-free whole grains.

A Healthy Plate

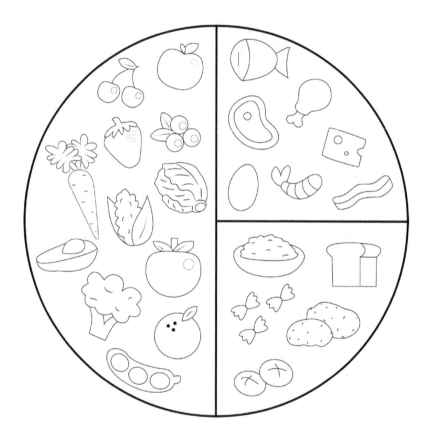

Seeds and Nuts: Seeds and nuts make wonderful snacks as they're loaded with the healthy, omega-3 fatty acids that your body craves and needs. (I'll talk about the importance of fats in Chapter 12.) Enjoy almonds, cashews, and macadamia nuts, along with sunflower and pumpkin seeds, raw, roasted or however you like them best. Unsweetened nut butters are perfect for snacking too.

Anti-inflammatory foods are high in fiber and aid in the production of butyrate (butyric acid), which is good for digestion and helps in the restoration of intestinal tissue. Butyrate is created by the fermentation of good bacteria feeding on dietary fibers in your gut. Every time you eat high fiber foods, like asparagus, artichokes, onions, bananas, apples, carrots, oats and potatoes, your colon produces more butyric acid.

TAKE PROBIOTICS

Remember when I told you that three factors have to be present in order to get celiac disease? You must have one of the two celiac genes, you must be eating gluten, and you must have some sort of intestinal permeability or leaky gut episode. When these three factors are present, your body is ripe for disease, and that is when celiac disease rears its ugly head.

When I was first diagnosed with celiac disease, I had no idea that my gut health was in shambles and that the bacteria in my gut was compromised in any way. I simply followed my doctor's orders and implemented a strict gluten-free diet with the hopes that I would *eventually* feel better. However, after complaining to my friend about how my bloating and gas persisted long after I'd broken up with gluten, she suggested that my gut health might be in bad shape and recommended that I take a daily probiotic supplement.

Believe it or not, at the time I was skeptical about taking a probiotic because I knew little about gut health or nutrition. I was desperate to feel better, so I decided to give her suggestion a try. Within a day, I started to feel better, and in a few days, I felt a lot better. My gut health went from *chronically gassy and bloated* to feeling *fine and dandy.*

While a lot of research has yet to be done on the role of probiotics in gut and whole-body health, millions of people, like me, have experienced the power of probiotics firsthand. This is why I think they are worth trying when you have a gluten disorder or any sort of autoimmune condition.

WHAT ARE PROBIOTICS?

Probiotics are living microorganisms of bacteria and yeast that are sold as dietary supplements and taken orally. While you might think of bacteria as harmful, the truth is that good or *beneficial* bacteria are essential for maintaining good health, nutrition and immunity.

Microorganisms live all over and inside our bodies. There are more than one thousand species of bacteria living on your skin alone, trillions of microbes living in your gut, and more than 1,000 different species of bacteria in and around your body. In fact, most humans are carrying around five pounds of bacteria at all times.[88]

Unfortunately, there is not a lot of specific science on the benefits of probiotics, and the U.S. Food and Drug Administration (FDA) has not approved probiotics for preventing or treating disease. That said, there is mounting evidence that demonstrates the role of creating and maintaining good gut health and a healthy microbiome, all which can be helped via probiotic supplementation.

In patients with celiac disease, the mucosa (small intestine lining) is damaged, which is accompanied by altered gut bacteria and increased intestinal permeability (leaky gut). Several studies suggest that celiac patients have reduced levels of bifidobacteria and lactobacilli, and that many celiac patients are unable to reestablish ideal gut microbiome on their own; they would therefore benefit from the addition of beneficial bacteria via probiotic supplementation.[89] [90] Another study found that in many celiac patients, "microbial imbalances persist in spite of a strict gluten-free diet" and that probiotics "might be of help in controlling gluten-mediated inflammation and ameliorating clinical symptoms."[91]

FINDING MR. RIGHT PROBIOTIC

To get the most out of your probiotic, first talk with your healthcare provider to get the clearance; then follow these guidelines:

Take a Probiotic Daily: It doesn't matter what time of day you take it. I prefer taking my probiotic before bed each night.

Take a High-Quality Probiotic: I take a potency of 50 billion CFUs for daily maintenance. CFUs stands for colony forming units or how much bacteria are in the probiotic supplement. If you're starting a probiotic regimen and your gut health is in shambles, ask your health care provider if it's okay to start with a dosage of 80-100 billion CFUs for 60 days. Then you can move to a maintenance routine of 50 billion CFUs or less daily.

Look for Bacteria Diversity: Look for brands that offer a variety of strains of bacteria. Switch brands often to introduce new strains of beneficial bacteria in your gut. Buy what's on sale and switch brands often to create bacteria diversity.

Refrigerated or Shelf Stable?: It doesn't matter if your probiotic is refrigerated or shelf stable, but if you buy refrigerated probiotics, they must stay refrigerated at all times.

Make Sure It's Gluten Free: Most brands I've seen at the grocery store are free from gluten, however, it's always wise to check labels for gluten ingredients and to never assume.

Avoid Probiotic-Laced Foods: Probiotic-marketed "health" foods include probiotic drinks and juices, as well as sugary yogurts. Most of these foods are loaded with sugar, and sugar is what feeds the bad bacteria in your gut. While you may be putting good bacteria in via supplementation, you'll also be feeding the bad bacteria their favorite food (sugar). Sugar is the exact food that helps the bad bacteria proliferate. This defeats the purpose of eating foods with probiotics in them in the first place.

Most commercially sold yogurts only contain one billion CFUs, a miniscule amount of good bacteria needed to help you restore your gut health. After consulting with your healthcare provider, I recommend taking 50 billion CFUs daily to get the biggest bang for your buck. You can easily get this amount in a supplement, but you'd have to eat an awful lot of yogurt to get even close to this amount of beneficial bacteria in your diet.

Try Fermented Foods: A great way to boost the beneficial bacteria in your gut is to enjoy fermented foods like kimchi, sauerkraut, or homemade fermented pickles. My personal favorite fermented food is kombucha, which is a fermented tea beverage. Kombucha tastes like fizzy soda and is loaded with healthy yeast and bacteria. It may not sound appetizing, but it tastes sweet even though it contains very little, if any, sugar. You can buy kombucha at most grocery stores, or make your own by following my step-by-step instructions at: goodforyouglutenfree.com/making-your-own-kombucha/.

NO MORE *SWEET* TALKING

Those bad bacteria have big egos and want to rule your gut. Care to guess which food bacteria crave most? It's sugar!

If you've ever baked bread, you know that you first combine warm water, yeast, and sugar in a bowl and let it sit for a few minutes until you see the mixture froth and bubble. When this happens, you benefit from a visual clue alerting you to the fact that the yeast is active and blooming (if you don't see bubbling, your yeast is old and dead). You know what made that yeast bloom and dance? Sugar.

Now imagine that unwanted yeast was alive and well in your gut and then you ate a bunch of sugar. Can you visualize the yeast and bacteria blooming inside your gut as it does when you're getting ready to bake bread?

Unfortunately, bacteria dysfunction in your gut can lead to all sorts of other gut disorders, including a common one known as candida albicans. Candida is an aggressive buildup of yeast that colonizes in your small intestine. As the sugar-eating yeast grows, it tries to break free by creating tiny holes in the intestinal lining, allowing bits of food particles to enter, or "leak," into your bloodstream. In other words, when unwanted yeast and bacteria proliferate in your gut, you end up creating a new source of leaky gut without ever taking another bite of gluten.

Researchers first implicated candida as a trigger for celiac disease. As yeast builds up in your small intestine, it can lead to intestinal permeability, and cause the celiac disease gene(s) to "turn on" in genetically predisposed individuals.[92] Additionally, another study found that 33 percent of people with celiac disease also had candida while no one in the control group had it, concluding that cases of candida are "significantly higher" in people with celiac disease.[93]

You should always talk to your doctor if you experience persistent gastrointestinal symptoms. Your doctor is the only one who can diagnose candida. He or she might prescribe an antifungal medication to give you some relief, but what works best in the long run, and what will prevent candida in the future, is to starve the yeast of sugar, its food source. It's a slow slog to recover from candida, and some sufferers experience flu-like symptoms as the yeast slowly dies off.

Similarly, a buildup of unwanted bacteria in the gut can lead to another gut disorder called small intestinal bacterial overgrowth (SIBO). This disorder means bad bacteria are setting up shop in your small intestine and making it challenging for you to evict them. Like candida, SIBO can create lingering, gut-wrenching symptoms long after you've ditched gluten. One study found that 18 percent of newly diagnosed celiac disease patients may have SIBO, which can contribute to persistent symptoms that mimic unmanaged celiac disease.[94]

SIBO is treated in a number of ways. For example, your doctor may prescribe an antibiotic. The problem is that, in many cases, SIBO returns, and there is little evidence to suggest that antibiotics work in treating the disorder long-term.[95] It's most important to identify the underlying cause of SIBO and then intervene with nutritional therapies that address the root cause. For those with gluten disorders, strict adherence to the gluten-free diet is a must, as is limiting sugar and carbohydrate consumption.

If you're suffering from continued poor gut health, consider laying off sugar-laden foods in order to starve and kill off the icky yeast and bacteria that have set up residence in your gut. Don't make your gut hospitable to these foes, or they'll never want to leave.

KNOW THY SUGARY SOURCE

Sugar is found in carbohydrates like flour, bread, grains, dairy products, electrolyte beverages, and cereals.

Sources of sugar and artificial sweeteners to beware of include:

- Agave syrup
- Aspartame
- Molasses
- Beet sugar
- Brown sugar
- Cane sugar
- Caramel color
- Cane juice
- Coconut sugar
- Confectioner's sugar
- Cornstarch
- Corn syrup
- Date sugar
- Destine
- Dextrose
- Equal
- Fig syrup
- Fruit juice
- Fructose
- Glucose
- Granulated sugar
- High fructose corn syrup
- Honey
- Invert sugar
- Lactose
- Mannitol
- Modified food starch
- Monosaccharides
- Polysaccharides
- Powdered sugar
- Raw sugar
- Rice syrup
- Saccharine
- Sorbitol
- Sorghum syrup
- Splenda
- Sucrose
- Sweet'N Low
- Turbinado sugar
- Xylitol

It's wise to lay off artificial sweeteners in addition to natural sugars. It's been well-documented that diet drinks and artificial sweeteners make you crave more sugar (and gain more weight), and that artificially sweetened foods and beverages are counterproductive to your healing.[96] On top of that, I've never seen a study that suggests one can overcome a sugar addiction – or lose weight – by switching from sugar to artificial sweeteners. If such a study exists, big food companies would have made sure you know about it.

As you limit or eliminate sugar from your diet in order to heal your gut, cravings for sugary foods may intensify. The bacteria and yeast may gnaw at you, demanding that you feed them. You would act desperately, too, if you were being starved to death! When the sugar cravings escalate, have some easy-to-grab snacks ready (that contain low to no sugar) to get you over the hump, such as salted and/or roasted nuts, an apple with a nut butter spread, fresh-cut vegetables (cucumbers, celery and carrots are personal favorites) with hummus, smashed avocado with lime and salt, olives, roasted chickpeas, roasted seaweed snacks, a fresh vegetable and fruit smoothie, and/or beef or turkey jerky.

10 Tips to Curb Your Sugar Cravings

1. **Avoid Packaged Foods:** Most packaged foods are loaded with white refined flour and added sugars. Instead, eat foods that are whole and fresh like avocados, berries, and sliced veggies.

2. **Avoid Sugary Sodas and Energy Drinks:** These "beverages" are what I like to call sugar delivery systems. A 20-ounce bottle of Gatorade contains 34 grams of sugar. A can of Coke contains 39 grams of sugar. These two drinks are equal sugar offenders. Don't be fooled by marketing hype.

3. **Avoid Artificial Sweeteners:** As mentioned, artificial sweeteners just make you crave sweet foods. Avoid them.

4. **Enjoy a Savory Breakfast:** Most people start their day with cereal, bagels, waffles or toast, and all of these foods are made with white refined grains that convert to sugar. They then top their waffles (sugar) with syrup (more sugar) and enjoy it with a side of orange juice (even more sugar!). When we start off our day with sugar, we crave more sugar as the day progresses. This is why if you're serious about curbing your sugar cravings, I recommend starting your day with a savory breakfast like scrambled eggs topped with salsa and sliced avocado, or sautéed veggies with turkey bacon.

5. **Eat Sweet Vegetables:** If you crave something sweet, enjoy sweet vegetables like carrots, sweet potatoes, beets, corn, onions, and squash. These vegetables offer the sweetness you crave along with the fiber and nutrients you need to heal.

6. **Enjoy Fruit in Moderation:** While fruit contains natural sugars (fructose), it also comes perfectly packaged with the essential nutrients and fiber your body needs to process the sugar. Your liver will metabolize most of the fructose whereas glucose (which comes from added sugar) will immediately begin circulating in your blood and spike your blood sugar.[97] This is why fructose has the lowest glycemic index rank of all sugars.

   If you're struggling with your gut health, and perhaps have candida or SIBO and are looking to starve out the sugar, consider eating mostly low-sugar fruits until you feel better. Low-sugar fruits include berries (raspberries, blackberries, blueberries, strawberries), kiwi, peaches, grapefruit, melons and avocados. Once your gut balance is restored, you can and should again enjoy all fruits as they are loaded with nutrients and fiber your body needs to heal.

7. **Read Labels:** By now you are an efficient label reader, ready to sniff out gluten in anything. Now take a moment to carefully examine nutrition labels and ingredient lists for sources of sugar. Condiments, salad dressings, coffee creamers, and yogurts all contain sugar. A container of flavored Yoplait yogurt, touted as a probiotic-rich food, contains 27 grams of sugar and, of the 170 calories, 108 come from sugar. Eater beware.

8. **Eat Whole vs. Refined Grains:** Gluten-free whole grains such as quinoa, brown rice, millet, and buckwheat slowly digest in your body compared to white, refined grains that rapidly convert to sugar. Limit white refined starches like white rice, white breads, potatoes, and cereals, and instead enjoy a small serving of whole grains each day to

help you feel full longer without adding excess sugar to your diet. If your gut issues persist, consider cutting out all grains – even gluten-free whole grains – until your symptoms resolve.

A Note About Bread: Whole grain breads are often touted as healthy, but when it comes to sugar, it doesn't matter if the slice of bread is whole wheat, whole grain, or gluten free, it ranks high on the glycemic index, spikes your blood sugar, and is happily feasted on by the bad bacteria residing in your gut.

It's best to avoid eating bread until your candida or SIBO symptoms subside. However, if you love bread and find it hard to resist (as I do), please enjoy whole grain bread in moderation, or consider trying gluten-free sourdough bread. Sourdough bread contains a probiotic bacteria known as lactobacillus, which, as we've discussed, supports gut health. Sourdough bread also has a lower glycemic index than whole grain bread.[98] There are tons of recipes online that will show you how to make a gluten-free sourdough starter and bread of your own, however, if you prefer to buy sourdough, a company called Bread SRSLY ships loaves of gluten-free sourdough throughout the U.S.

9. **Drink Up:** When you're hungry or craving sugar, drink a glass of water with a lemon squeeze or muddled cucumber. We often mistake thirst for hunger or cravings. I find that a glass of water helps me feel full and deters me from reaching for something sweet. Kombucha can also satisfy that sugary beverage or soda craving as it's fizzy and sweet despite containing little or no sugar.

10. **Learn to Cook at Home:** Get back to basics and learn to cook at home (and love cooking at home, too!). Avoid eating an excessive number of your meals out of the house where you have little to no control over how much sugar – and gluten – is put into your food. Avoid fast and cheap food like the plague. The more you can plan your meals,

the less likely you will reach for something sweet and fast. Visit goodforyouglutenfree.com/dear-gluten-resources for a free one-week, low-sugar meal plan.

THE PACKAGED FOODS CONUNDRUM

Unfortunately, what passes for "food" these days often isn't really food. Food scientists have created a lot of Frankenfood in an attempt to make food irresistible and addictive. Packaged foods have become a breeding ground for a slew of unsavory ingredients including preservatives, food dyes, fillers, artificial flavors, sugar, GMOs, and more.

This is why you must not fall into the gluten-free packaged foods trap. Of course it's helpful to know there are tons of gluten-free packaged products to help make our lives easier (which they do), but be forewarned that eating excessive packaged foods is one of the main contributors to poor health outcomes such as weight gain and disease. Just because a product is labeled "gluten free" says nothing about whether or not it's healthy or good for you. In fact, as we just discussed, foods made with wheat substitutes like rice, corn, tapioca, and potato starch still spike your sugar load.

Unfortunately, many people with celiac disease and gluten sensitivities find themselves gaining weight on the gluten-free diet. I've been there myself. When a friend brings me a gluten-free donut, I eat it. However, I rarely ate donuts before I went gluten free, so I often wonder why am I eating this donut now? Is it because I don't want to hurt my friend's feelings, after she was so thoughtful to get me a gluten-free donut? Is it because I feel deprived and wonder when I will have access to a gluten-free donut again? This gluten-free business really messes with your brain! On top of that, as a gluten-free blogger, I sometimes justify eating the donut in the name of research.

I've learned over the years that eating gluten free shouldn't be a license to eat as many gluten-free donuts as I want if I'm determined to maintain a healthy weight and lifestyle. I have to remind myself to "back away from the donuts" or just eat them every so often, as a treat.

For you, I suggest using your break-up with gluten to change your habits for the better. Use and eat packaged foods infrequently – like when you want to enjoy the occasional sweet treat, or when you need an emergency meal (or snack) because there's nothing safe for you to eat. Don't become dependent on packaged foods for your everyday meals and snacks, or your waistline may grow while your health continues to deteriorate.

EAT ORGANIC

You may have heard about the benefits of eating organic foods, but perhaps you don't know why or the full story. I'd like to share a bit about how genetically modified organisms (GMOs), and the chemicals sprayed on today's crops, just *might* be contributing to your poor gut – and whole body – health, thereby inhibiting your body's ability to fully heal from your gluten disorder.

THE DOWNLOAD ON GMOS

Americans consume an estimated 193 pounds of genetically engineered foods per person each year.[99] The problem is that genetically modified foods *may* be linked to illness in our country. GMOs are engineered by powerful biotech companies, including Monsanto, a company that also manufactures and sells weed-killing glyphosate (marketed as Roundup™). Unfortunately, according to the Non-GMO Project website, there is no "scientific consensus" related to the safety of GMOs, and there have been no epidemiological studies on the impact of GMOs on human health.

There are nine genetically modified crops currently being produced: Soy, corn, cotton (oil), canola (oil), sugar beets, zucchini and yellow squash, potatoes, Hawaiian papaya, and alfalfa. Scientists have either deleted or inserted genes into these crops to make them pesticide-resistant.

Wheat is not (yet) classified as a genetically modified crop; rather, wheat has been crossbred and hybridized over thousands of years, creating dramatic alterations and shifts in its genetic structure. As a result of crossbreeding and hybridization, thousands of known strains of wheat are commercially produced, none of which has been tested for potential ill-effects on the humans who consume them.

ARE YOU GONNA EAT THAT GLYPHOSATE?

While wheat is not genetically modified, per se, some wheat growers, as well as many farmers who use genetically modified seeds, use glyphosate to aid in crop management and larger yields. In 2016, 33 percent of wheat acres in the U.S. used glyphosate.[100] The World Health Organization even classified glyphosate as "probably carcinogenic."

When you eat a genetically modified piece of produce, you are eating something that was likely sprayed with glyphosate. Glyphosate kills all the bugs and weeds, but it doesn't kill the crop. Why? Because GMO seed manufacturers have genetically modified crops to resist weed and bug-killing chemicals. The problem is that the weed-killing glyphosate residue remains on your apple even after you attempt to wash it off, and then you eat it without knowing what those bug-killing chemicals are doing to your gut or health.

I understand why farmers love glyphosate-resistant seeds; such products grow better because they're not being ravaged by bugs and weeds. Farmers enjoy high yields when they spray their crops with chemicals without harming the produce itself. GMO technology even saved the Hawaiian papaya from extinction.[101] However, I have no idea how GMOs, or the chemicals sprayed on these chemical resistant crops, are impacting my microbiome. Could either GMOs or the chemicals sprayed on GMO crops be contributing to my intestinal permeability (leaky gut)?

THE CASE FOR ORGANICS

I buy organic produce as much as possible. Organic-labeled products prohibit the use of GMOs and glyphosate, along with a long list of other prohibited substances. You can also look for Non-GMO Project verified products when shopping for packaged foods.

I realize that eating organic can be expensive, especially if you're on a tight budget and have a big family to feed. If you can't buy everything organic, consider buying *some* products organic. The Environmental Working Group (EWG) puts out a list every year that features what it calls the Dirty Dozen. These are the dozen fruits or vegetables that, when tested by the EWG, contained the most pesticide and chemical residue. Strawberries, peppers, leafy greens, peaches, and celery continually top the Dirty Dozen list, which you can view at EWG.org. Anything on that list should be purchased organic, when possible. The EWG also has a Clean 15 list noting the produce that tested with the least chemical residue.

If your gut is compromised by years of eating gluten, there's no need to continue to assault it with bug- and weed-destroying chemicals. If these chemicals kill weeds and bugs, imagine what they might be doing to the delicate lining of your gut. Remember, the goal is to heal, not to continue to set off Molotov cocktails inside your small intestine.

USE ONLY MEDICALLY NECESSARY ANTIBIOTICS, WHEN NEEDED

A contributor to dysbiosis in your gut may come from the over-consumption of antibiotics. When you take an antibiotic, you obliterate all the bacteria, good and bad, in your gut. Studies have shown that in two years post-antibiotic usage, a person's microbiome is still not back to normal. Don't get me wrong, antibiotics can be life-saving and/or symptom-relieving medications when used properly; it's when they are overused that we get into trouble. Remember, 70 percent of our immune system is in our gut; and when we wipe our guts clean of all bacteria, good and bad, we make ourselves prone to illness.

Unfortunately, we are not only exposed to antibiotics through medications, but also through the foods we eat. Animals are given the majority of antibiotics in the U.S., and they're mostly given antibiotics prophylactically to prevent disease from spreading among animals living in close quarters. I personally don't want to consume products from animals pumped with antibiotics, so I buy organic meat and dairy where animals are administered antibiotics only when they are sick.

Antibiotics, unfortunately, are becoming more commonplace among farmers who are spraying it on their crops (including rice!) to prevent insect infestations, fungal diseases, and bacterial infections. Researchers found that this potentially harmful agricultural practice is being done "far more frequently and on a much greater variety of crops than previously thought," exposing humans to unnecessary antibiotics when we consume these crops.[102] Fortunately, organic practices prohibit the use of antibiotics.

IT TAKES GUTS! NICHOLE THOMAS TAKES A HOLISTIC APPROACH TO WELLNESS

Nichole Thomas, a former Syracuse University basketball player and the wife of former NBA star Etan Thomas, had been "sick" for as long as she can remember.

Thomas suffered from chronic stomach aches, severe bloating, brain fog, memory and focus issues, plus infertility. She had been variously diagnosed with disorders such as ADD, depression, chronic fatigue syndrome, fibromyalgia, lupus, and Hashimoto's thyroiditis.

The list of *"things wrong with her"* was long and complex, but none of these diagnoses or their subsequent treatments provided her with any relief. Thomas was left feeling frustrated; she desperately wanted answers to what was behind her seemingly endless list of symptoms.

In 2008, Thomas decided to take her mom's advice and visit a naturopath. A naturopath is professionally trained to help individuals heal through natural interventions. The naturopath ran a few tests and discovered Thomas had a "severe" wheat allergy. She immediately recommended Thomas remove wheat, and all products that contain gluten, from her diet and skin care products.

"It felt like someone removed the veil from my face. I not only felt better without gluten but also my fertility issues were suddenly resolved, and I was pregnant with our third child in just a few weeks after starting the gluten-free diet," she says.

IS IT CELIAC?

Eight months after Thomas was diagnosed with a wheat allergy, she thought it would be wise to get tested for celiac disease. However, when she learned that in order to be tested for celiac, she would need to eat gluten for several weeks (see Chapter 2 and the Gluten Challenge), she decided against the testing.

Instead, she took a DNA test, which uncovered that she had both HLA-DQ2 and HLA-DQ8 genes. Both genes meant she was at high risk of having celiac disease, and that she likely inherited the genes from both her mom and dad.[103] In light of her genetic markers and symptoms, her doctor diagnosed her with celiac disease.

A FAMILY AFFAIR

As a result of her DNA test, Thomas suspected her mom and dad might also have celiac disease and that they both were carriers of the gene. Each had unique symptoms that suggested gluten might be the culprit.

At the time, her father was suffering from late stage kidney disease and congestive heart failure. The doctors had given him six months to live and told him his kidneys would never heal.

Thomas didn't agree with the dire diagnosis. "I told him your body *will* heal if you give it a chance, and I recommended he eat gluten free," she recalls.

Her father agreed to give the gluten-free diet a chance; and three years later, against all odds, was feeling great and his kidney function rebounded from 19 to 60 percent. (Thomas notes that years later, in 2018, her father went on a gluten binge and later tested positive for celiac disease.)

Thomas' mother, at the time, was suffering from painful rheumatoid arthritis (RA). Thomas recommended she ditch gluten, which she did, and within no time she felt better. Through an elimination diet, her mother also discovered that corn flares her RA symptoms. Her mother now eats corn-free as well and is completely off all of her RA medications with specific doctor's orders to "keep doing what you're doing."

"It's fascinating and heartbreaking to think that so many people are dying prematurely because they have these food sensitivities, and they just don't know," she laments. "This is especially true in the African-American community, where information [about celiac disease and food sensitivities] is not top of mind in doctors' offices and testing is not readily available."

HOLISTIC HEALING

Thomas says her grandmother used to tell her, "Wisdom is lived experiences." These are words that Thomas says she lives by to this day.

"The process of healing isn't just about removing gluten; rather, it requires a holistic approach. It's learning to listen to what your body is telling you and acting on the cues it sends you," she says. "Only when I began to eat better foods, take supplements, rest more, and nourish my body did I begin to feel better."

In addition to healing physically, Thomas adds that she worked on her emotional and spiritual healing too. "I needed to give myself a little grace. I used to beat myself up for being depressed and not having a lot of energy to do everything I wanted to do, but once I started to focus on wellness, I came to realize that my depression was only a symptom of celiac disease. It wasn't really who I was."

Today, Thomas lives a gluten- and sugar-free life. Her daughter has gluten sensitivity too. Now the entire Thomas family eats gluten free.

"I have real compassion, empathy and understanding of what people are going through. Their suffering resonates with me, and I understand it because it *was* a part of my life once, too," she says.

Chapter 11
REST YOUR DIGESTIVE SYSTEM

"The food we take into our mouth goes into our stomach, where it gets digested and eventually assimilates into the bloodstream. Our blood is what creates our cells, our tissues, our organs, our skin, our hair, our brains and even our thoughts and feelings. We are, at our most basic level, walking food."

– Joshua Rosenthal

Before I knew I had celiac disease, I would wake up feeling amazing. My stomach was flat, and I felt healthy and ready to start the day anew, skinny jeans and all. But, as the day progressed, I gradually felt worse. My stomach would begin its daily journey to bloat up like a balloon, and by the end of the day, I looked six months pregnant and I'd have to unbutton those skinny jeans or risk popping a seam! Then, overnight, my belly would miraculously flatten and I'd feel great again, resetting the vicious bloating cycle for the day. Why did I feel skinny and light in the AM, but bloated and heavy in the PM?

This led me to a major aha moment. When my digestive system rested, it restored itself; when it was working hard to digest the food I was eating, it bloated up like a balloon. I wondered if I could find ways to rest my digestive system for longer periods of time, and, if by doing so, I could accelerate the restoration and healing that my gut desperately needed.

If I broke my leg, I would rest it as much as possible, right? I wouldn't plan a hike or go for a long walk. I'd use my leg only when I had to until it fully restored and healed. I decided to apply this same logic to my "broken" gut. Instead of using my digestive system all day long and zap it of its energy, I would instead reserve that energy for repairing and restoring.

Following are resting strategies that worked for me and I hope they work for you too. Give them a try and see if a little vacation is all your broken digestive system needs to rejuvenate from its daily stressors.

GET INTO GREEN JUICING

Years ago, a friend of mine told me one of the best ways to rest my digestive system and flood my body with the nutrients it so desperately needed was to drink green juices. To this day, I believe green juicing changed my life for the better. For many months post-celiac diagnosis, I made myself a daily green juice (or purchased a cold-pressed green juice at the store), and I'd enjoy it as a snack or meal replacement. Even today I still enjoy a green juice, albeit more occasionally now that I've healed and eat plenty of fresh vegetables each day, something I rarely ate in my pre-celiac days.

Digestion begins in the mouth. As you start chewing and breaking down your food, your saliva assists by making digestive enzymes that aid in the breakdown of the food. The food goes on to your stomach where it is broken into even smaller bits before it makes its way into your small intestine for further processing.

However, when you break down your food before putting it in your body, the juicer or blender is doing part of the heavy lifting for you, making the nutrients more readily available for your body to process, maximizing your nutrient load, and resting your digestive processes. You don't have to chew all those vege-tables, nor fire up the digestive mechanisms in your stomach, to break down large bits of food. In fact, your body doesn't have to lift a finger to soak in all that anti-inflammatory goodness. Juicing makes it easy for your body to quickly absorb all those *good for you* nutrients.

While juicing (or blending) is a great way to load up on vegetables and fruits while resting your broken digestive system, it also offers a few other benefits that aid in your healing process. First, it strengthens your immune system, and you may find that you get sick less, which lowers your need for antibiotics and medical interventions. You may also find you have more energy, feel lighter, have better skin, hair and nails, and are able to think more clearly.

Additionally, juicing fills you up. This means you'll naturally crowd out foods from your diet that offer little nutritional benefit, and you might also kickstart weight loss as you reduce cravings for sugary foods and load up your body with nutrient-dense foods instead.

Finally, juicing may help you live longer. A study published in the *New England Journal of Medicine* found that people who added more fruits and vegetables to their diet over time improved their chances of living longer.[104] Cheers to that. Now drink up!

Visit goodforyouglutenfree.com/10-amazing-juicing-recipes to get started with juicing and download 10 delicious juice recipes.

LIMIT SNACKING

Another strategy to resting – and thereby restoring – your digestive system is to limit snacking. I used to snack all day long, especially if someone left cookies in the breakroom at work. I had no idea, at the time, that by snacking often, I was keeping my digestive juices firing on all cylinders at all times. However, by limiting the amount of snacks I enjoyed, and by focusing on eating more nourishing meals that kept me full longer, I was not only able to give my body time to digest each meal without overloading my digestive system, but also I was giving it a chance to rest between feedings.

AVOID OVEREATING

A lot of people with celiac disease struggle with overeating. This is because we're used to eating and eating and not truly feeling nourished. You might call someone with celiac disease well-fed but undernourished. I would eat often because I always felt hungry, and I later learned this was because I was nutrient deprived. My body had no way of knowing it was truly satiated because it was unable to completely absorb all the nutrients from the food I was eating. I wasn't hungry; my body was telling me to eat because it lacked nutrients, not food.

Once I broke it off with gluten, I continued to overeat because, as the old adage goes, old habits die hard. I had to train myself to eat until I was full, and I had to be careful not to overstuff my digestive system with excess food that it didn't need.

Overeating not only taxes your digestive system, but it can also cause you to gain weight and feel sluggish. If your digestive system is working hard, other systems in your body will run slow too. It's like having too many windows open on your computer at one time.

Tune into your body's signals. Stop eating when you feel nearly full. Doing so will prevent a bottleneck of food from queuing up in your digestive tract, and it will avoid making your already taxed digestive system work overtime to process excess food.

CHEW YOUR FOOD

It's extremely important that you chew your food thoroughly. Not only does chewing mechanically break down your food, but also, your salivary glands release digestive enzymes that aid in the chemical breakdown of your food too. The more enzymes released (via chewing), the less pressure is placed on your digestive system to break down these large particles of improperly chewed food.

LIMIT HARD-TO-DIGEST FOODS

Some foods are easier to digest than others, and when your digestive system is in shambles, it's wise to limit eating foods that are difficult to digest.

One of the foods that can be difficult for your body to properly digest is meat and animal products. It takes a lot of digestive juices to properly break down meat into digestible bits. One of the strategies I've employed in my post-celiac world is eating what I call veggie-forward meals. This means I eat smaller portions of meat at each meal (or go meatless several nights a week), and instead load up on plant-based proteins and vegetables.

Other foods that are difficult to digest include fried foods, sugar (and artificial sugar), highly processed foods, and dairy.

DRINK BONE BROTHS

Bone broth can be a healing tonic that soothes the digestive system, cools the inflammatory fire in the gut, and offers nutrients that restore and strengthen the intestinal lining of your gut. When made properly, bone broth offers a variety of vitamins, trace minerals, and collagen (a protein that contains amino acids essential for strengthening your bones, connective tissues, and skin) to your nutrient-deprived system.

A good bone broth is made by simmering either chicken, beef, or fish bones for 8-24 hours in water. You then remove the bones and drink the remaining broth. I recommend using only organic chicken, beef, or fish bones for added healing benefits.

HEALING CHICKEN BONE BROTH RECIPE

Ingredients:

- 2-3 lbs. chicken parts (bones, feet, backbone, neckbone, wings, and/or legs)
- 4 quarts cold filtered water

- 2 tbsp. apple cider vinegar
- 1 large onion, coarsely chopped
- 2 carrots (peels left on), coarsely chopped
- 2 celery sticks, coarsely chopped
- 1 bunch parsley
- 2-inch ginger or turmeric root (optional)
- Kosher salt, to taste

Directions:

1. Place boney chicken pieces in a large stainless-steel pot with water, vinegar, and all vegetables except parsley.
2. Bring mixture to a boil and remove any scum that rises to the top.
3. Reduce heat, cover, and simmer for 8-24 hours. The longer you cook the stock, the richer and more flavorful it will be.
4. About 1 hour before finishing the stock, add parsley. This will impart additional minerals into the broth.
5. Remove large chicken pieces with a slotted spoon. If there is meat on the bone, remove and use the meat for other dishes or in the soup upon serving.
6. Strain the stock into a large bowl and reserve in your refrigerator until fat rises to the top and congeals, usually overnight.
7. Skim off the fat and discard. Reserve the stock in covered containers in your refrigerator or freezer.

Note: You can purchase organic chicken bones (without meat) from many grocery stores. Talk to your local butcher. You can also use a whole cut-up chicken and simply save the meat for the soup or other dishes. Additionally, you can use leftover bones from roasted chicken (or rotisserie chicken) as the bones for your broth. Roasted bones will add depth to your broth.

EVALUATE ANTACID INTAKE

Now that you're resting your digestive system, avoiding gluten, and eating a mostly anti-inflammatory diet, your stomach probably won't need to work as hard to break down food. This means if you've suffered from heartburn or acid reflux in the past, you may not suffer from it anymore. The foods that once made your stomach acid bubble up in discomfort are a thing of the past.

On top of that, you want to have fully functioning stomach acid, and antacid and proton pump inhibitors impair your production of hydrochloric acid or stomach acid. Your digestive system desperately needs hydrochloric acid to properly break down your food. Without it, undigested food particles will make their way into your small intestine, and may tear through your delicate intestinal lining, "leak" out of your gut and into your bloodstream, and cause inflammation at weak links in your body.

If you currently take antacids or proton pump inhibitors, talk to your doctor about making a plan to reduce and eventually eliminate these drugs. Your need and dependency on antacids will likely change as your diet changes, and your body needs fully functioning stomach acid to properly break down and digest your food from here on out.

EMPLOY INTERMITTENT FASTING STRATEGIES

Many people have successfully used intermittent fasting as a way to rest their digestive system, improve their health, and shed a few unwanted pounds of fat in the process.[105] Intermittent fasting is when you go through periods of eating and then periods of fasting. While I am far from an expert on this topic, I would like to recommend you investigate intermittent fasting as a health-promoting exercise in your life, especially if your digestive health has been compromised and you're struggling to feel well.

There are a few simple ways to incorporate intermittent fasting into your life without feeling like you're starving. An easy way is to simply limit or eliminate snacking. When you do this, you will give your body 4-5 hours between eating breakfast, lunch and dinner, as well as a long break between dinner and breakfast.

Another way to incorporate intermittent fasting in your life is to fast for 12 hours every day, which I do myself. I don't typically eat between the hours of 7pm and 7am. I simply eat my dinner and then allow my digestive system to rest for 12 hours, giving my digestive system time to restore and regenerate during this 12-hour window. One study found that participants who fasted for a 12-hour period were better able to burn stored fat cells, release toxins, and lose weight.[106]

I have found intermittent fasting to be rewarding. I don't find myself mindlessly eating before bed anymore. After I eat my dinner, I brush my teeth and close the kitchen for the night. I am generally in my pajamas by 7pm, signaling to my body that I'm ready to rest... and digest!

DIGESTIVE TLC

Giving your digestive system much-needed time to rest and restore requires you to change deep-seated habits. You may not be used to eating vegetables, or you might be a big snacker or night grazer. Challenge yourself to try new things. Maybe start with juicing and see how you feel, then gradually move on to intermittent fasting, and/or eating less meat and more vegetables. Build on each new practice and see what works for you. I had no idea I would love juicing so much and it's become a well-worn habit I employ even today, eight years into my celiac journey. Every step you take to nourish your body is a step in the right direction, and the process of healing is a marathon, not sprint. Go easy on yourself, implement things at your own pace, and remember, you don't have to do it all. Experiment with various techniques and see what "sticks" for you.

CHAPTER 12
SUPPLEMENTING YOUR HEALTH

"The food you eat can be either the safest and most powerful form of medicine or the slowest form of poison."

– Ann Wigmore

D id you know that nearly 90 percent of newly diagnosed celiac disease patients have one or more nutritional deficiencies?[107] This is not surprising given that gluten has destroyed the lining of the small intestine, an organ essential for nutrient absorption and distribution.

While you can obtain most of the nutrients you need from the food you eat, some supplementation can aid in and accelerate your healing and help you (re)build your immune system more quickly. Supplements alone are not enough; they must be taken in conjunction with a health-promoting diet. Be sure to discuss adding supplements to your diet with your healthcare provider.

VITAMIN CHECK

I was fortunate enough to have a doctor who thought to check my vitamin levels after my celiac diagnosis. This is where I first learned I was depleted in many essential nutrients, particularly vitamins B and D. I have since learned that it is no longer standard practice to check vitamin levels as some insurance companies have deemed vitamin checks no longer medically necessary. This is despite the fact that half of the worldwide population has a vitamin D deficiency.[108]

Fortunately, if your doctor or insurance company refuses to test your vitamin levels, there are several at-home vitamin test kits available that enable you to check and monitor your vitamin levels yourself so you can ensure you're where you need to be. Visit goodforyouglutenfree.com/dear-gluten-resources for the latest information on these tests.

While I'm not an expert on supplements, I have done research and experimentation with a few common supplements that have aided me on my healing journey. I'd like to share what I've learned with you and encourage you to do your own research and talk to your healthcare team about whether these supplements could help accelerate the healing in your body, too.

VITAMIN D

Vitamin D plays a crucial role in your overall health. It aids in the absorption of calcium to ensure strong, healthy bones. It also plays a starring role in your digestive health. In fact, evidence suggests that vitamin D helps regulate inflammation in your gut and helps create a healthy microbiome.[109]

I suggest consuming vitamin D-rich foods and a vitamin D supplement to ensure you get plenty of it, as every cell in your body needs it. While vitamin D-rich foods are rare, good sources include fatty fish (salmon, sardines, tuna), eggs, and soy milk or almond milk fortified with vitamin D.

Beyond food and supplementation, a good source of vitamin D comes from spending some time in the sun each day. Just 15 minutes of sun every afternoon can do wonders for your health as vitamin D is absorbed through the skin from sunlight. Just be sure to allow the sun to coat your arms and legs. Of course, don't let yourself burn; apply sunscreen when exposed to excessive sun.

You'll still soak in enough of the sun's ultraviolet B (UVB) rays while protecting your skin from sun damage.

VITAMIN B12

A vitamin B12 deficiency is common in celiac disease patients, with one study finding that 41 percent of untreated celiac disease patients suffer from low levels of vitamin B12.[110] This is because gluten impairs a celiac disease patient's ability to properly absorb nutrients from the foods he or she is eating. Even if you're eating vitamin B12-rich foods, which are typically found in animal products (meats, poultry, eggs, milk, etc.), your body is still not able to process those nutrients properly.

Subsequently, a vitamin B12 deficiency can lead to a slew of annoying and damaging symptoms. Most commonly, a lack of vitamin B12 can lead to low energy or chronic fatigue. Other symptoms of a vitamin B12 deficiency include anemia, weakness, dizziness, pale or yellowed skin, diarrhea or constipation, numbness, soreness of the tongue, and various brain dysfunctions such as depression or confusion.

Once you break up with gluten, your body will slowly but surely begin to properly absorb vitamin B12 again; supplementation will ensure you're getting the amount you need and may help remedy your symptoms faster.

FOLIC ACID

Folic acid, or B9, is another B vitamin that our bodies use to make new cells, including the mucosal cells that line the small intestine and replace themselves every week. One study found that a large number of newly diagnosed celiac disease patients (20 percent) were deficient in folic acid.[111] Folate is a naturally occurring source of folic acid and is found mostly in leafy green vegetables such as kale, spinach, asparagus and Brussels sprouts. It is also found in avocados, beans, fortified cereals, citrus fruits, eggs, and animal products.

Because most Americans don't eat enough leafy green vegetables, and to reduce the risk of birth defects in newborns, which has been tied to a folate deficiency, the FDA requires manufacturers to add folic acid, a synthetic form of folate, to breads, cereals, flours, corn meals, pastas, rice, and other grain products. Gluten-free foods are made from a combination of grains and starches, and therefore contain less folic acid than their gluten-full counterparts.[112]

The best way to get folic acid is still via natural food sources. However, adding a multivitamin that includes folic acid to your daily supplement intake can help ensure you're getting enough. Talk to your doctor about the right dosage for you.

FISH OIL

On top of boosting your intake of vitamins you've likely been deprived of for so long during your relationship with gluten, another supplement that I consider essential to your health is a fish oil supplement.

Fresh, fatty fish can be a welcome addition to your gluten-free diet as it's naturally gluten free, and fish contains plenty of omega-3 fatty acids or essential fats that your body needs. Our body thrives when it's fed a healthy serving of "good" fats each day.

Before we talk about what kind of fish oil supplement you should take, I'd like to briefly discuss the role fats play in our diet. Both omega-3 and omega-6 are essential fatty acids found in everyday foods we consume. Our bodies cannot make these fatty acids, so it's essential we consume them. Unfortunately, Americans overconsume omega-6 fatty acids as they're commonly found in corn and vegetable oils used to cook fast food and junk food. When we consume too many omega-6s and not enough omega-3s, well, Houston, we have a problem.

Unfortunately, few people consume enough omega-3 fatty acids to counterbalance the overconsumption of omega-6s, making fish oil supplementation, a good source of omega-3s, an important part of a healthy living regimen.

The major benefit of taking a fish oil supplement is its role in deterring inflammation. Fish oil contains DHA (docosahexaenoic acid) and EPA (eicosapentaenoic acid), which are known for their anti-inflammatory properties. DHA and EPA are beneficial to your brain (your brain is 70 percent fat!), heart health, and have been shown to lower inflammation and chronic disease.[113] In fact, one study found that an omega-3 supplement had the "equivalent effect" of reducing arthritis pain as ibuprofen in patients with acute and chronic nonspecific neck and back pain.[114]

When purchasing a fish oil supplement, look for one that contains low levels of mercury. If the ingredient list contains tuna, put it back on the shelf as tuna contains some of the highest levels of mercury contaminants. You don't want to create inflammation in your body while you're trying to fight it. Low-mercury fish found commonly in high-quality fish oil supplements include anchovy, cod, herring, krill, sardines, and salmon. As with all supplements, be sure to consult your healthcare provider to determine the proper dosage for you.

MYTH-BUSTING! DOES FAT MAKE YOU FAT?

Many people mistakenly associate eating fat with getting fat, but quite the opposite is true. Our bodies don't need a lot of carbohydrates to thrive; rather, our bodies need fat for energy and fuel. A low-fat diet impairs one's ability to burn calories, and one researcher found that subjects on a low-fat diet burned 325 fewer calories per day than patients on a high-fat diet.[115]

Don't believe me? In 1992, the U.S. government encouraged a high-carb, low-fat diet, later endorsed by both the American Heart Association and American Diabetes Association. Guess what happened as a result of this diet "wisdom?" The number of people who became diabetic and obese in the following years surged, and this number continues to skyrocket today as the low-fat myth continues to run its course. In fact, in the early 1960s, only 13 percent of adults were classified as obese; by 2018, 42 percent of adults were classified as obese.[116] The numbers don't lie.

Fight Free Radicals (aka, Oxidative Stress)

Our bodies contain free radicals, which are waste products from various toxin exposures that bind to and eventually damage our cells. Free radicals come from the foods we eat and the air we breathe, as well as from sources such as infections, tissue damage and radiation. The best way to fight free radicals is by consuming plenty of antioxidant-rich foods. In fact, you could say antioxidants are the antidote to oxidative stress.

Antioxidants work by gobbling up free radicals floating around in your body, just as Pac-man gobbles up pellets. However, trouble brews when our bodies have more free radicals than antioxidants to gobble them up. When this happens, a phenomenon known as oxidative stress occurs.

Oxidative stress is a figurative "browning" or aging that happens inside of you. After you cut into an apple and leave it exposed to air, you can see it start to brown. This same oxidation happens inside you when free radicals pile up in your bloodstream. In fact, too many free radicals, and too little antioxidants to gobble them up, can lead to inflammation, cell damage and disease. Researchers have found oxidative stress levels to be even higher in gluten-sensitive patients than the general population.[117]

You can stop or at least slow down the figurative "browning" inside of you by consuming plenty of antioxidant-rich foods like berries, cherries, leafy green vegetables, green tea, coffee, and my personal favorite, dark chocolate (in moderation, of course). You can also take an antioxidant supplement as extra insurance against oxidative stress. I personally take a daily supplement that contains antioxidant-rich ingredients including milk thistle, bacopa, ashwagandha, green tea, and turmeric.

Replenish Your Nutrient Bank

Gluten has impaired your body's ability to properly absorb nutrients, and it's likely you've been suffering from nutrient deprivation for years. This is why I believe a diet rich in antioxidants, healthy fats, and plenty of vitamins D, B12, and folic acid, will help replenish your nutrient bank and support you in creating and maintaining good health.

Remember, food should always be your first source of nutrient-dense fuel; however, proper supplementation can help you more quickly replenish your depleted nutrient tank, keep it full, and keep disease at bay.

CHAPTER 13
WHAT ELSE COULD IT BE?

*"Trust your intuition. You don't need to explain
or justify your feelings to anyone; just trust your
own inner guidance, it knows best."*

– Anonymous

C hances are that once you implement the gluten-free diet
and clean up your diet from gluten-free junk food, you
will feel better. However, you may break up with gluten
and still feel lousy. This means something more might be at play.

In this chapter, I'd like to discuss what else might be holding
you back from experiencing your best, healthy self. Could there
be more to your failing health than just gluten?

CROSS-REACTIVITY

If your body is unresponsive to the gluten-free diet, you might
be experiencing what is known as cross-reactivity. This is when
a food causes your immune system to respond in a similar way
to how it responds to gluten. Your body is programmed to make
antibodies to toxins and foreign substances, and unfortunately
it can become confused by proteins that look similar to gluten.

Your body may start producing antibodies to what it perceives as a toxin, even if it's a *normal* food.

Foods that have been known to create cross-reactivity in some people with celiac disease or gluten sensitivity include dairy, oats, corn, rice, and yeast.

Casein, for example, is a protein found in dairy and has a similar molecular structure to the gliadin protein found in gluten. Your body might confuse the two proteins, causing your immune system to go into attack mode just as it does when it detects the presence of gluten. This may be why a lot of people who don't tolerate gluten also cannot tolerate dairy. In fact, almost 50 percent of people with celiac disease also have an intolerance to cow's milk.[118]

To know if your body is reacting to a specific food, you can either eliminate the food from your diet for four weeks, then slowly reintroduce it to see how you feel, or you can take a blood test to help you identify cross-reactive foods to gluten. One such test is the Cyrex Array 4 gluten cross-reactivity test from Cyrex Laboratories. Talk to your doctor if you want to get to the bottom of why your symptoms haven't completely resolved despite being on a strict gluten-free diet.

FOOD SENSITIVITY

Beyond cross-reactivity, you may also have one or more additional food sensitivities. Maybe after eating eggs you experience bloating, gas, and abdominal pain, and/or non-digestive symptoms like migraines and fatigue. This might mean you have a food sensitivity to eggs.

It's important to distinguish that a food sensitivity is not a food allergy. A food allergy test is looking for what foods or toxins cause your body to produce IgE antibodies (vs. IgG antibodies). A wheat allergy, for example, is a food allergy that is very serious and impacts 0.4 percent of the U.S. population. Some food allergies, like a peanut allergy, can be life-threatening and should be taken extremely seriously.

However, food sensitivity is still a bit uncharted in the medical world, and many food sensitivity tests are considered controversial. A food sensitivity test looks for how the IgG antibodies bind to each food and by what degree. IgG accounts for 70-75 percent of the antibodies circulating in your blood.[119] Antibodies are an important part of your body's response to toxins because they recognize and bind to particular antigens, such as bacteria or viruses, and then help destroy those toxins.

When a food sensitivity test picks up on dozens of high reactivity foods, it may not mean you're reacting to all those foods; it may instead mean you're eating those foods and suffer from leaky gut. The test is finding IgG antibodies left and right because so many foods are leaking out of your gut and into your bloodstream. In fact, a food sensitivity may simply be indicative of the foods you're eating most vs. foods that are bothering you.

Before taking a food sensitivity test, first put in the hard work to repair and seal your leaky gut. Once your gut is healed, a food sensitivity test may find that you're still reacting to one or two foods now. Those are foods worth eliminating from your diet. Eliminate the top reactive foods (the ones with the highest IgG ranking on your test) for four weeks. Then, slowly over time, reintroduce each food and see how you feel. You will likely know, at this time, which foods bother you and which do not. Continue to eliminate and reintroduce foods until you get to the bottom of what is ailing you most. You are your best detective. No one can figure this out but you. Food sensitivity tests just give you a starting point as to which suspect foods might be at the root of your symptoms.

I took an at-home food sensitivity test after I put in the hard work to heal my gut. It came back with no high reactive foods and only a few moderate reactive foods, including almonds, watermelon and cottage cheese. I ate a lot of almonds so I decided to eliminate almonds from my diet and the dull tummy pain I had disappeared. I realized, perhaps, I was eating too many almonds and products that included almonds. After four weeks of eliminating almonds, I modestly reintroduced them to my diet and felt fine. Today I eat almonds, but I do so only in moderation. It was when I was eating them in excess that they were creating stomach woes for me.

FRUCTAN INTOLERANCE

Many people with self-diagnosed gluten sensitivity might actually have a fructan intolerance vs. gluten sensitivity. A fructan is a carbohydrate found in wheat and some vegetables. Fructans are oligo- or polysaccharides that include short chains of fructose units. (Fructans comprise the "O" in FODMAPs, which stands for fermentable oligosaccharides, disaccharides, monosaccharides and polyols.)

What you need to know is that humans lack the digestive enzymes needed to break down oligo- or polysaccharides. In fact, we absorb only 5-15 percent of the fructans we consume and the rest is sent to the colon to be naturally fermented. This can lead to gas and other digestive woes in some people, and such symptoms are often confused with gluten sensitivity.

While fructans are most commonly found in products containing or made from wheat, such as breads, pasta and couscous, they are also found in barley and certain vegetables such as onions, shallots, scallions, garlic, Brussels sprouts, cabbage, broccoli, pistachio and artichokes.

Researchers found that fructans – more so than gluten – induced bloating and other gastrointestinal symptoms in individuals with self-reported non-celiac gluten sensitivity.[120]

If you suspect you have a fructan sensitivity, your doctor can give you a breath test, although be forewarned that the results are not always reliable. You can also eliminate all sources of fructans from your diet for four weeks to see if you feel better.

Remember, not all fructans are "bad." In fact, if you're not sensitive to them, they offer a good source of soluble fiber and help you maintain a healthy blood sugar level. They also serve as prebiotics, which feed the beneficial bacteria that reside in your digestive tract, which promotes overall health.

HORMONE IMBALANCE

Hormones impact gut function and gut function impacts hormones. Any sort of imbalance can lead to a variety of annoying gastrointestinal symptoms including but not limited to leaky gut, bloating, gas and diarrhea.

The birth control pill is one of the key contributors to this hormonal imbalance in women. According to Dr. Jolene Brighten, in her book, *Beyond the Pill*, the pill is a known contributor of a slew of health consequences including but not limited to digestive tract inflammation, increased risk for autoimmune diseases, thyroid and adrenal malfunction, high cholesterol and blood pressure, and nutritional deficiencies, all which can lead to anxiety, depression, mood swings and other brain disorders. In fact, she says there is a 300 percent increase in the risk of developing Crohn's if you take the pill.[121] I can't help but wonder if all those years (15 years to be exact) of mindlessly taking the pill elevated my risk for developing celiac disease.

Beyond birth control, it is well-known that antibiotics, environmental toxins, undiagnosed food sensitivities, and poor diet may all contribute to hormone imbalances, which can be addressed by changing your diet and minding – and mending – your gut health. If you continue to feel unwell despite eating gluten free, take a closer look at your hormone health and talk to your doctor about how you can work towards naturally restoring and balancing your hormones, even if that means getting off the pill.

ENVIRONMENTALLY ACQUIRED ILLNESS

The International Society for Environmentally Acquired Illnesses says that it is "likely" that the epidemic of unexplained chronic disease may be caused, at least in part, by increased exposure to toxic chemicals present in our food supply and via environmental irritants.[122]

In fact, long-term exposure to mold in your home or office (often referred to as "sick building syndrome") has been linked to a slew of chronic disorders including but not limited to autoimmune disease, celiac disease, gluten sensitivities, leaky gut syndrome, Alzheimer's, Parkinson's, cancer, depression, psoriasis and eczema.[123] A May 2020 study found that children and young adults who were exposed to endocrine-disrupting chemicals found in pesticides, nonstick cookware, and fire retardants had a higher risk for celiac disease.[124]

Your doctor can test you for mold exposure via a blood test that looks for antibodies your body makes to different mold species. If you find through testing that you have mold toxicity, you'll need to identify the source of mold in your home or office, and take steps to remediate it.

Your risk of mold toxicity increases if your home or office has ever experienced flooding, if you're regularly exposed to chemicals at work, if you have mercury dental fillings, and/or if you live in a high pollution area.

If you suspect you have an environmentally acquired illness, talk to your doctor, or, even better, find a specialist to help you. A list of physicians who specialize in environmentally acquired illnesses can be found at https://iseai.org/find-a-professional/.

STRESS

Stress is a known trigger for celiac disease, and stressful events, including pregnancy, often precede a celiac disease diagnosis.[125] Additionally, stress can impair your body's ability to heal from celiac disease and other gluten disorders. In fact, stress hormones have been known to weaken and damage your gut lining, alter gut bacteria, contribute to a leaky gut, and make your body prone to disease. Ninety percent of all serotonin, a hormone that helps transmit messages between nerve cells and is critical to modulating mood and digestion, is made and stored in your gut.[126]

When you're chronically stressed, your body constantly craves sugar because it needs glucose to keep you moving at an intense level. Your body uses glucose for energy and stores about 2,500 calories of it to help you in times of intense stress. For example, if a bear is chasing you, your body will need to initiate its fight-or-flight response, tapping into the glucose to help you muster up all the adrenalin you need to (hopefully) outrun the bear. Unfortunately, it doesn't take a bear chasing you to activate your fight-or-flight response these days. Sitting in traffic, a high-stress job, or a stressful relationship can cause your body to tap into its glucose reserves and put you in a chronic state of stress.

Consider this: If you're stressed out, and your body is burning glucose all day long, what do you think your body will crave? You guessed it, your body will need you to replenish its glucose reserves and refuel your adrenaline tank. This means you'll crave sugary foods over and over again.

If you continue to live in a state of stress, you'll continue to activate your body's stress response and you'll continue to crave sugar. As a result, you'll probably gain weight because you're only burning sugar, not fat, you won't be able to sleep, and things like your skin, hair, nails, and digestive system take second fiddle and start to deteriorate.

PHYSICAL SIGNS YOU'RE LIVING IN A CHRONIC STATE OF STRESS

- Bloating and gas
- Brittle hair or nails
- Chronic colds and infections
- Chronic fatigue
- Constipation
- Frequent sweating
- Headaches
- Intense sugar and caffeine cravings
- Trouble sleeping
- Mood swings
- Skin issues
- Rapid heart rate
- Loss of sexual desire

On the other hand, when you're living a low-stress lifestyle, you are living in what is commonly called the "rest and digest" state where your parasympathetic nervous system functions at an optimal state. When your body is at rest, all your energy can be diverted to helping your behind-the-scenes functions perform optimally. Your hair and nails can grow. Your blood can pump. And your digestive system can digest. Your body burns fat vs. glucose, proving that stressing less actually promotes weight loss!

If you're still experiencing gut issues despite being on a gluten-free diet, consider the role of stress in your life. How can your body properly digest its food when all your energy is being put towards constantly outrunning the proverbial bear? No amount of kale or probiotics will heal your digestive ailments if you're constantly burning the midnight oil (glucose).

When I was diagnosed with celiac disease and as I experienced persistent digestive woes, I took a hard look at how I was living my life and searched for ways I could stress less and tap into my parasympathetic – or *rest and digest* – system. Here are a few strategies that worked for me:

Limit Caffeine: Caffeine is a stimulant that activates your sympathetic nervous system, keeping you in a state of go-go-go! Take a look at your relationship with caffeine and how it might be affecting – and putting unneeded stress – on your body. Is there a way you can limit how much caffeine you consume? I used to drink caffeine every morning, but found that it was making me jittery. After several months of weaning myself off caffeine, I am proud to say that I only consume caffeine on occasion now. I like the taste of coffee, so every morning you'll find me sipping on decaf coffee instead.

Work Less: Your health depends on getting a grip on your work schedule and ensuring it's not the source of chronic stress in your life. Learn to say "no" without apology when something doesn't fit in your busy schedule. Schedule down time. Never feel bad about doing what's best for you and your health, even if it means moving at a slower-than-usual pace.

Set a Sleep Schedule: Sleep is essential to good health, particularly good digestive health. When you sleep, your body goes into its "rest and digest" phase. I realize, however, that sleep is fleeting for so many people. Stress, poor health, and/or a hormone imbalance, for example, can contribute to difficulties falling or staying asleep. The good news is, that as your body heals now that you've split with gluten and you're working towards improving your health, it's likely your sleep will improve as well. Prioritize sleep in your life by going to sleep at a regular time each night and waking up at the same time the next morning. Allow yourself 7-8 hours each night to sleep. If you struggle to fall asleep, audit your pre-bedtime routine. Are you working? Watching TV? Or are you reading, meditating or doing another relaxing exercise? Remember, as your body heals, chances are your sleep will improve. Sleep is restorative, particularly for your digestive system, so don't skimp on sleep.

Live Clutter Free: I believe a cluttered space is the sign of a cluttered mind. Keep your work spaces and home free from clutter, especially your bedroom. The bedroom is no place for your home office, and never store clutter under your bed. You don't want to be literally sleeping on top of clutter, do you? Regularly dispose of items that are no longer serving a purpose in your life. Practice Marie Kondo's art of tidying up. When an item is no longer of use to you, thank it for the role it once played in your life and let it go.

Rid of Negative Energy and People: If something (or someone) is constantly stressing you out, find a way to remove it (or him or her) from your life. I like to hang out with people who are positive and calm, and I keep my distance from those who are negative and constantly bring the drama.

Practice Calming Exercises: You can counteract stressors with calming daily activities such as meditation, reading a book, or taking a walk. Scientists have found that such calming activities actually change your brain function and cell expression.[127] If you have a stressful work or home life, consider countering the stress with calming exercise vs. high intensity workouts. Do whatever you can to put your body in a stress-free zone so it can function optimally.

Get Physical: Physical fitness is a great immunity booster. Exercise can help you get and stay healthy and quickly bounce back from colds and viruses. It's also a proven stress reliever and can boost those feel-good, post-workout endorphins.[128] Your body works well when it's being physically challenged. Walk or bike daily, go to an aerobics class (is it okay to admit I love Jazzercise?), or start a gym membership and actually go! The more you put into taking care of your body, the faster it will heal and thrive. Even patients recovering from surgery are on their feet shortly after their procedure because doctors know that movement and exercise is an essential component to a speedy recovery.

Be Social: Being social and interacting with others is an essential part of healing and living a low-stress life. Having friends and meaningful relationships reduces stress and increases the production of your happiness hormones such as endorphins, dopamine, and serotonin. You can still enjoy time with friends and family even if you need to make adjustments to *how* you do it in order to accommodate your gluten-free lifestyle.

NON-RESPONSIVE OR REFRACTORY CELIAC DISEASE

Non-responsive or refractory celiac disease is a serious condition experienced by people with celiac disease whose symptoms related to malabsorption and damaged villi persist despite being on a strict gluten-free diet for 6-12 months. Only 1-2 percent of the celiac disease population will develop refractory celiac disease; it is most commonly found in people over the age of 50, and rarely found in children.[129]

The symptoms of refractory celiac disease are similar to those of celiac disease, however, they can often be more severe and debilitating. For people with type 1 refractory celiac disease, aggressive nutritional therapies, strict adherence to the gluten-free diet, and other medical and pharmacological interventions may improve one's prognosis. However, in more difficult cases, or type 2 refractory celiac disease, many patients develop T-cell lymphoma, a rare form of cancer, and prognosis is poor, with a five-year survival rate of 40-58 percent.[130]

Again, refractory celiac disease is very rare. Most people with celiac disease find that their bodies are responsive to the gluten-free diet, and they're able to put their symptoms into remission. However, if symptoms persist despite eating a strict gluten-free diet for 6-12 months, please consult your doctor.

CHAPTER 14
THE SILVER LINING

"Life appears to me too short to be spent nursing animosity or registering wrongs."

– Charlotte Bronte

S aying goodbye to gluten and healing physically and emotionally is not for the faint of heart. It has taken me years to arrive at a place where I feel comfortable grocery shopping, eating out, advocating for myself, and feeling my best, healthy self again.

There are, however, many positive outcomes that come from breaking up with gluten, many of which you might only be able to "see" in hindsight. It's hard to see the big picture – the silver lining – when you're in the thick of dealing with a disorder that more-likely-than-not has turned your life upside-down.

The truth is, I believe celiac disease happened *for* me, not *to* me. That is why today I live with gratitude – not resentment – for celiac disease.

While leaving gluten was challenging and difficult in many ways, I see it as a gift. I no longer take my health for granted, and I'm actively looking for ways to make my health better. If I hadn't been diagnosed with celiac disease, I believe I was well on my way to having additional life-challenging and threatening ailments, and perhaps even dying young.

I equate being diagnosed with celiac disease to being rerouted by my personal global positioning system (GPS). Celiac detoured me from the ill health that lay ahead, and rerouted me in the right direction. Knowing I had celiac disease, and knowing I could do something about it, allowed me to change the trajectory of my health for the better. I worked hard to heal my body, and I continue to work hard to maintain good health and deter disease in my life. While I do have fears about the future and what will become of my health, right now I am living life to its fullest. In fact, I believe I have figured out how to stave off disease in my life in ways I may have never known how to do had my health not been shaken to its core by celiac disease. Every day I am healthy is a true gift.

I'm also thankful that my health can be helped by diet, and I'm not dependent on drugs or surgical procedures to prolong my life. By eliminating a specific food, I'm showing myself self-love and am working hard at being healthy. I take no prescription pills and the only over-the-counter medication I take is an allergy pill to relieve my hay fever symptoms. Unfortunately, nearly half of the U.S. population is on some sort of prescription medication – for blood pressure, acid reflux, thyroid issues, diabetes, depression, etc.[131] I take none.

I see so many people suffering and dependent on medications to help them get through the day. I don't say this to make anyone feel bad about needing prescription drugs, but I do take solace in knowing that I was able to deter these diseases in my life. Without knowing I had celiac disease, and catching it early, I was well on my way to falling apart. Will I always be free of prescription drugs? I cannot say for sure. I only know, since I was diagnosed with celiac disease eight years ago, and as a 43-year-old woman, I am dependent on none. I employ true "health" care in my life.

Furthermore, I have made so many new and wonderful friends *because* of the gluten-free diet. These are the people who have come into my life *because* of celiac disease, those who have made my life richer and fuller. We are bonded by a disease, diet, and friendship for life. We uniquely know what one another is going through. We revel in new restaurant finds and in helping each other in ways I've never had friends help me before.

Also, celiac disease has given me the gift of seeing my husband in a new and wonderful way. After watching me struggle to eat gluten free in this cruel world desensitized to the plight of the gluten-free eater, and after realizing how lonely and isolating it must feel, he decided that our entire kitchen would be gluten free and that he would go gluten free too. He stood in solidarity with me. If it happened to me, it happened to him. What a beautiful way to show me just how much he loves me! And, as a bonus result of going gluten free, my husband's thyroid, which was creeping towards hypothyroidism, normalized. A win-win for all. I have never felt so supported and loved by my life partner. Celiac disease gave me this extraordinary insight and gift.

The gluten-free diet has also brought out the best in so many supporters in my life. My mother-in-law always makes gluten-free meals for our Friday night family dinners and has become quite the gluten-free chef. My friend Rochel Goldbaum hosted a holiday gathering and made everything gluten free *because* of me. She told me, "If you're eating at my house, you get to eat everything." She even made gluten-free donuts to show me how important I am and so I wouldn't feel left out come dessert time. This stood in dark contrast to the prior night when I went to another friend's house and the only gluten-free option for the entire evening was a fruit salad even though, when I spoke with her in advance, she told me there would be "plenty" of gluten-free options. (Don't worry, I didn't starve. I, of course, brought my own emergency stash of food because you must always be prepared.)

My kids, too, have become much better human beings *because* of my celiac disease. While they don't have to eat gluten free, they are protective of me. My 12-year old daughter has become quite the supportive little mama in my life. This winter, after a long day of skiing, we found ourselves waiting in a huge line at Chipotle in Silverthorne, Colorado. When I saw the line, I announced to my family that I didn't want to be a bother by asking the staff to change gloves and get me fresh ingredients. This would hold up the line even more, and I would feel bad for doing so. I decided, instead, that I would just get chips and guacamole. When I told my family my plan, my daughter gave me a serious pep talk. She told me I deserved to eat a full meal, too, and I should never feel bad about asking for a safe meal. She pushed me to ask the staff to change gloves and get me fresh ingredients, even though I would hold up the line, and threatened to do it for me if I didn't speak up. Of course, as it turns out, the staff didn't mind helping me at all; they are used to "allergy" orders. It perhaps took an extra minute to make my burrito bowl; and at the end of the day, it was no big deal. Sometimes we need the love, support, and encouragement of others to get through the daily struggles of being on the gluten-free diet. Sometimes I need someone to be my voice of reason, to push me to do the right thing.

Finally, I'm grateful celiac disease can be helped by diet and is not terminal if managed properly. This makes fighting to get a gluten-free meal seem a little less challenging when I put things into perspective. Mind you, no one's suffering is greater than another's. When the suffering happens to you, it's very real and raw. I am, however, able to see that I have control over my suffering, and it all comes down to what I put in my body.

Is eating gluten free easy? Never. It is and most likely always will be a daily struggle for me and for you. It's a burden we bear, a challenge given to you and me. I cope as best as I can, and sometimes I allow myself to have a pity party for one. It's in these times when I'm grateful that chocolate is gluten free. So is ice cream.

In the end, I must thank Gluten for giving me these gifts and allowing me to go on living a life full of health rather than disease. Our relationship has been complicated, but now it's done. It's over. We're through. Like I said before and I'll say again, Gluten, it's not me, it's you. And in the apropos words of Ariana Grande, "Thank you, next."

Chapter 15
You Are Not Alone

*"The secret to staying young is to live honestly,
eat slowly, and lie about your age."*

– Lucille Ball

Chances are, somewhere along your journey, you will encounter naysayers and people who resist your shift to get healthy. You'll find people who tell you, "A little gluten won't hurt you," or "Green juicing is just a bunch of hooey; you don't really believe that?!?" and you must, at all times, stay the course through such resistance.

It's not uncommon for such resistance to cause self-doubt and fear. Always remind yourself that you are on your own healing journey. What works for you, and what you intuitively know works for you, may not work for others nor be someone else's cup of tea. The only person you have to answer to is you. This is why I encourage you to steer clear of negative people, naysayers, and doubting healthcare providers. There are other fish in the sea who will offer a positive word of encouragement, or lend a supportive ear.

You are not and will never be alone on your journey to become gluten free and healthy. There are millions of us following a gluten-free diet who are here for you!

CELIAC ORGANIZATIONS

If you live in a big city, chances are there is a local celiac disease or gluten-free diet support group near you. Search the National Celiac Association website – nationalceliac.org/celiac-disease-support-groups – to find a local support group.

If you don't have a support group near you, create your own. Meetup.com is a great tool for starting a support group, and social media can help you find others seeking friendship and support from people who share the gluten-free lifestyle.

You can also find support online wherever you are in the world. I facilitate the Gluten-Free Diet Support Group on Facebook – facebook.com/groups/GlutenFreeDietSupport. I regularly pop into the community to answer questions, decode ingredient labels, share restaurant recommendations, and vent frustrations.

And of course, look for guidance from an expert – a physician, nutritionist, dietician, and/or health coach – who specializes in gluten disorders and functional or integrative medicine. These professionals can guide you through your messy breakup with gluten and help you achieve the health and lifestyle you desire.

NEVER STOP LEARNING

In addition to finding support on the ground and online, I encourage you to learn more about gluten disorders. Knowledge is power. Hopefully, I have whetted your appetite to learn more, and now you're anxious to continue to seek out ways to improve your health and heal your body.

Here are some books I highly recommend:

The Autoimmune Fix by Dr. Tom O'Bryan
Wheat Belly by Dr. William Davis
Undoctored by Dr. William Davis
Grain Brain by Dr. David Perlmutter
The Ultramind Solution by Dr. Mark Hyman
Beyond the Pill by Dr. Jolene Brighten
Hashimoto's Protocol by Dr. Izabella Wentz

Food Matters by Mark Bittman
How Not to Die by Dr. Michael Greger

FREE RESOURCES

Visit goodforyouglutenfree.com/dear-gluten-resources to download the following resources:

- Download the *Dear Gluten Cookbook*, which includes 20 gluten-free recipes exclusively curated for *Dear Gluten* readers.
- Download a sample 7-day gluten-free meal plan, and my guide to meal planning.
- Download a free copy of my printable Gluten-Free Safe Dining Card

... and so much more!

CAN YOU HELP?

Did this book help you? If so, please share it with others by leaving me a review on Amazon.com. Your simple gesture will ensure that others struggling to break up with gluten will be able to find the important information they need to finally call it quits with gluten and improve their health and lives for good. Thank you!

XO, Jenny

PART III

THE RECIPES

Moving On

Nothing heals a broken heart like moving on with some delicious new (comfort) foods you can easily make and enjoy safely at home. Your relationship with gluten may be over, but your love affair with food has only just begun...

My Food Philosophy

The gluten-free diet isn't a diet at all. It's a lifestyle. My goal is to help you get healthy without feeling deprived or like you're on a diet.

I believe you should be able to enjoy bread, cakes and cookies as long as you balance those indulgences with a variety of *good for you*, anti-inflammatory foods.

My recipes are meant to bring normalcy to your life. You'll notice they're simple, straight-forward recipes using as many naturally gluten-free ingredients as possible, all while getting you to see how simple it is to cook and bake without gluten.

I have provided only a handful of my most favorite recipes next. Most of my recipes and the foods I eat every day are on my website, goodforyouglutenfree.com, and in my weekly meal plans. Visit goodforyouglutenfree.com/dear-gluten-resources for a downloadable seven-day meal plan you can try for yourself. My goal is and always has been to make eating gluten free as easy and tasty as possible.

Now I'd like to share some favorite recipes with you.

RECIPES

FAVORITE NON-BORING BREAKFASTS

CRISPY KALE WITH FRIED EGGS

If you love a savory breakfast that packs a nutritional punch, you'll love my sautéed kale and fried egg breakfast. Kale gets crispy when fried in a little oil whereas other leafy green vegetables, like spinach, turn soggy. Kale is also one of the most nutritionally-dense foods on the planet. Enjoy kale, alongside protein-rich eggs, to start your day with the energy and fuel your body craves.

Prep Time: 4 minutes
Cook Time: 12 minutes
Yields: 1 serving
Equipment: Medium non-stick pan

1 tbsp avocado oil (or other vegetable oil)
2-3 kale leaves, stems removed and leaves roughly chopped into bite-sized pieces
½ tsp butter
2 large eggs
Salt and pepper, to taste

Heat oil in a large pan over medium-high heat. Add kale leaves to hot oil and mix until leaves are evenly coated with oil. Continue to cook kale for 8-10 minutes until kale leaves begin to crisp, mixing occasionally. Season kale with salt and pepper (to taste) and add kale to a plate.

Return pan to stovetop and lower heat to medium. Add butter to the pan and once butter is melted, crack eggs and cook as desired. Top with salt and pepper, to taste.

Add fried eggs to the top of the crispy kale and serve immediately. Serve with a side of gluten-free toast (optional).

PROTEIN PANCAKE

If you love a warm, slightly sweet breakfast, give this gluten-free protein pancake recipe a try. It's a healthier version of traditional pancakes, and it boasts tons of energy-boosting fats and fiber to keep your digestive system running smoothly.

Prep Time: 1 minute
Cook Time: 4 minutes
Yields: 1 serving
Equipment: Small non-stick pan

1 large egg
2 tbsp water
1/3 cup quick cooking gluten-free oats
1 tsp flaxseed meal
1 tbsp honey
1/4 tsp vanilla extract
1/2 tsp ground cinnamon
1/4 tsp butter

In a small bowl, whisk egg and water together with a fork. Add oats, flaxseed meal, honey, vanilla and cinnamon and mix until well combined.

Melt butter in small skillet pan over medium-high heat. Once the pan is hot, pour the mixture into the pan and cook for about 2 minutes on each side until cooked through.

Top pancake with chopped fruit or simply enjoy it as is.

Easy Brussels Sprouts and Egg Breakfast Skillet

This simple, veggie-forward dish is perfect for breakfast (although I've been known to make it for lunch too). The Brussels sprouts caramelize as they cook, and the olives add a salty and tasty flare. Use pre-shredded Brussels sprouts to make this recipe easy-breezy.

Prep Time: 2 minutes
Cook Time: 15 minutes
Yields: 2 servings
Equipment: Large non-stick pan

1 tbsp butter, vegan butter, or avocado oil
12 ounces pre-shredded Brussels sprouts (about 4 cups)
3 garlic cloves, finely chopped
12 medium-sized green olives, chopped (about 1/2 cup)
4 large eggs
2 tbsp water
2 lemon wedges
Kosher salt, to taste
Fresh ground pepper, to taste
2 mini red peppers for garnish, optional

Melt butter in a large non-stick pan over medium high heat, then add shredded Brussels sprouts and cook for 7-8 minutes, stirring occasionally. The sprouts should soften and start to brown a bit on the bottom. Add garlic and olives and continue to cook for another 2 minutes.

Create four small wells inside the sprouts and gently crack an egg into each cavity. Add water and cover. Cook for 1-3 minutes until the eggs are cooked but still slightly runny. They yolks will grow a white skin on them.

Turn off heat, add salt and pepper to taste, add a squeeze of lemon, and garnish with slices of mini bell pepper. Serve immediately.

Tip! Swap Brussels sprouts for broccoli slaw instead. You can find packages of shredded broccoli slaw at most grocery stores.

FAVORITE CLASSIC DINNERS

BETTER THAN TAKE-OUT ORANGE CHICKEN

My favorite food group is Chinese food (lol!) but eating at most Chinese restaurants can feel like a contact sport. Most Chinese restaurants offer limited gluten-free selections, and there's always a risk of getting glutened.

When I'm craving Chinese food, I often find myself making my own Chinese take-out orange chicken. This recipe works well and gives you freedom to create your own sweet and sour chicken, lemon chicken, and/or pineapple chicken with a few simple swaps once you learn the basics.

Prep Time: 20 minutes
Cook Time: 10 minutes
Yield: 4-6 servings
Equipment: Large non-stick pan

Chicken:

1/4 cup avocado oil (or vegetable oil)
1.5 lbs boneless, skinless chicken breasts or tenderloins, cut into bite-sized pieces
1/2 cup cornstarch, more if needed
1 tsp kosher salt
1/2 tsp black pepper

Orange Sauce:

1/4 cup tamari or gluten-free soy sauce
1/2 cup water
1/4 cup freshly squeezed orange, approx. juice of one orange
1 tbsp orange zest (approx. equal to the zest of one orange)
2 tbsp white wine vinegar
2 tbsp brown sugar
2 garlic cloves minced (more if desired)

1/4 tsp red pepper flakes, optional (adjust to taste)
1 tbsp cornstarch

Heat oil in a large non-stick pan over medium-high heat. Combine cornstarch with salt and pepper in a medium bowl. Coat each piece of chicken in cornstarch mixture. Shake off excess corn-starch from each chicken piece and place into hot oil. Do not overcrowd the chicken. Bake in batches, if needed.

Allow chicken to cook for 2 minutes on one side before turning to cook the additional sides. Continue to cook chicken until it's evenly browned on all sides and the chicken is cooked through, about 8-10 minutes.

While chicken is cooking, combine all sauce ingredients in a small bowl and set aside.

Once chicken is cooked through (do not overcook), lower heat to medium and add sauce. Sauce will bubble and thicken. Continue to cook for 1 minute until sauce is thickened and each piece of chicken is fully coated. If the sauce is too thick, add more water (1/4 cup at a time), and continue to cook mixture over medium-high heat until sauce is to desired thickness. If the sauce is not thick enough, add a cornstarch slurry (1 tsp cornstarch mixed with 2 tsp water) to the mixture and stir well.

Remove from heat and top with sesame seeds and/or chopped green onions (optional) and serve over white or brown rice.

Variations:

(1) Swap orange juice and zest for lemon juice and zest
(2) Swap brown sugar for 2 tbsp of apricot preserves.
(3) Swap orange juice and zest for a can of pineapple chunks. Use the pineapple juice for the sauce, and add pineapple chunks to the final mixture just before serving.

Easy Chicken Tenders with Cilantro-Lime Cauliflower Rice

This easy weeknight meal is a staple in my house because, let's face it, who doesn't love chicken tenders? I fry the tenders in a large pan with oil, but you could spray the tenders with oil and then bake instead. Serve with cauliflower rice for a healthy treat, or use white or brown rice instead. Cauliflower is high in vitamins B6, C, K and folate, and is loaded with antioxidants that give your immune system a boost.

Prep Time:	15 minutes
Cook Time:	25 minutes
Yield:	4-6 servings
Equipment:	Large non-stick pan, food processor

For the Chicken:

3/4 cup gluten-free bread crumbs
1 tbsp Italian seasoning blend
½ tsp garlic powder
1 tsp kosher salt
Fresh ground pepper
1 egg
1 tbsp water
2-3 tbsp avocado or vegetable oil (more if needed)
2-3 organic chicken breasts, cut into long strips

For the Cilantro-Lime Cauliflower Rice:

Florets from 1 large cauliflower, stems removed and discarded
1 medium yellow onion
3-4 garlic cloves
1 tbsp avocado or vegetable oil
1 tsp kosher salt, to taste
2 lime wedges
¼ cup fresh cilantro, chopped

To prepare the chicken:

Combine bread crumbs, Italian seasoning, garlic powder, salt and pepper in a small bowl and whisk together. Set aside. In another small bowl, combine egg with 1 tbsp of water and mix well. Set aside.

Heat oil in a large non-stick pan over medium-high heat. Working in batches, dip chicken strips into egg wash, then coat the chicken with the breadcrumb mixture. Place each chicken strip into the hot pan. Do not overcrowd.

Cook chicken for about 3-4 minutes on each side until cooked through. Thicker pieces may take a bit longer to cook. If the outside of the chicken browns too quickly, lower temperature to medium heat.

To prepare the cauliflower rice:

Pulse a handful of uncooked cauliflower florets in your food processor 8-10 times, working in batches as to not overcrowd the food processor. The cauliflower should be finely chopped (like rice) but not mushy or fully blended. Set aside. Alternatively, use a bag of pre-riced cauliflower instead.

Roughly chop onion and add it to your food processor. Pulse until onions are finely chopped, approximately 8-10 pulses. Set aside. Add garlic cloves to the food processor and pulse 4-5 times until garlic is finely chopped. Set aside.

Heat oil in a large pan over medium-high heat. Add onion and cook for about 3-4 minutes until soft, then add garlic and riced cauliflower and continue to cook for 4-5 minutes until cauliflower is soft but not mushy. Add salt and stir well.

Turn off heat, stir in cilantro, and add lime juice, to taste.

Ridiculously Easy Refried Bean Rice Bowls with Corn Salsa

I always have a few quick and easy plant-based meals on hand for busy nights, and these refried bean bowls always hit the spot. I use canned beans, a pantry staple loaded with protein, fiber and lots of minerals like iron, magnesium, potassium and zinc. Look for canned beans with no sugar and low in sodium.

I don't drain my beans and instead cook the beans in their own juices. If you want to rinse your beans first, add about 1/2 cup of vegetable broth per can to your beans when cooking.

Prep Time: 20 minutes
Cook Time: 30-40 minutes
Yield: 6 bowls
Equipment: Rice cooker, medium stock pot, potato masher

For the rice:

2 cups brown rice
4 cups water
1 tbsp kosher salt
2 tbsp butter or oil

For the refried beans:

1 can black beans (do NOT drain)
1 can great northern white beans (do NOT drain)
1 tbsp chili powder
1 tsp ground cumin
1 tsp Kosher salt
Fresh ground pepper, to taste

For the corn salsa:

2 cans sweet corn, drained
2 red bell peppers, diced into small pieces

4 green onions (scallions), chopped into small pieces
1-2 tsp kosher salt, to taste
Ground black pepper, to taste
3-4 tbsp fresh chopped cilantro
2-3 lime wedges

Taco bowl fixings:

Avocado, sliced
Lettuce, shredded
Black olives
Shredded cheese, optional

To prepare rice:

Rice cooker (preferred): Combine rice water, salt, and butter or oil in your rice cooker and cook according to your rice cooker instructions.

Stovetop: Combine rice water, salt, and butter or oil in a medium pot and bring mixture to a boil. Cover, turn heat on low, and cook for 30-40 minutes until rice has soaked up all the water and is soft. Fluff with a fork.

To prepare refried beans:

In a medium sized pot, add canned beans, with juice, and turn heat to medium-high. Use a potato masher to mash and flatten the beans. They will get softer as they heat. Add chili powder, cumin, salt and pepper into the bean mixture. Continue cooking, while stirring often, until most of the liquid is cooked off, about 3-4 minutes after the mixture has come to a simmer. Turn off heat.

To prepare corn salsa:

Combine corn, pepper, onions, salt, pepper, cilantro, and lime juice, to taste, in a large bowl. Add salt, to taste.

Assemble your bowls:

Add rice to the bottom of a bowl. Top with refried beans, corn salsa, and all the taco bowl fixings as·desired.

HOMEMADE PASTA WITH AVOCADO PESTO SAUCE

My two-ingredient homemade pasta recipe has been one of the most popular recipes on my blog for several years and with good reason. We gluten-free eaters love our pasta, and rarely do we get the homemade stuff.

Once you master pasta-making at home, you can enjoy it topped with any sauce you desire. My kids love pesto sauce, so I've created a healthier, dairy-free version of this classic sauce, inspired by one of my favorite cookbooks, Oh She Glows.

Please note that if you don't want to go through the trouble of making your own gluten-free pasta, simply serve this recipe with store-bought brown rice pasta instead. Easy swap, right?

Prep Time: 30 minutes
Cook Time: 2-3 minutes
Yield: 4 servings
Equipment: Pasta machine (optional), food processor, rolling pin, large stock pot, food processor

For the pasta:

200 grams Bob's Red Mill 1:1 Gluten-Free Flour Blend (*see notes) + extra flour for dusting surfaces
3 large eggs

For the pesto sauce:

2 garlic cloves
1/4 cup fresh basil leaves
4 tsp fresh squeezed lemon juice
1 tbsp extra virgin olive oil
1 ripe avocado, pitted
1/2 tsp kosher salt
Fresh ground pepper, to taste
Lemon zest, for serving

Making the pasta:

Add flour and eggs to a food processor using the dough blade. Pulse about 12-20 times until a dough ball forms. Do not over-work dough. Remove dough from the food processor and place it on a lightly floured surface.

If dough is sticky, add a sprinkle of flour and mix it into the dough for 30 seconds until the texture is still wet but not sticky. Remember, gluten-free dough doesn't require kneading since there is no gluten to develop. If the mixture is too dry, wet your hands and play with the dough a bit to incorporate the water. You should be able to handle the dough without it sticking to your hands, and it should be wet enough so it doesn't crumble when handled.

Using your rolling pin, roll out dough into a thin flat layer on a floured surface or floured piece of parchment paper. Cut off and discard frayed edges. You can cut dough into strips using a pizza cutter (see notes below) or run sheets of the dough through your pasta machine. If using a pasta machine, run the sheets through the flattening/pasta sheet side, then run it through the pasta cutting side.

Boil a large stock pot with salted water (about 1-2 tsp kosher salt). When water is boiling, gently unravel pasta strands and add it to water. Do not overcrowd the pasta or it will clump. Cook for 1-2 minutes depending on the thickness of the pasta. Drain and rinse pasta with cold water. Serve immediately topped with pesto sauce or your favorite sauce.

For the pesto sauce:

Add garlic and basil to a food processor and pulse 10-12 times. Add lemon juice, oil, avocado flesh, and 1 tbsp water and process mixture until smooth, about 45-60 seconds. Season with salt and pepper to taste. Mix with pasta and top with lemon zest (optional).

Notes:

*If your gluten-free flour blend doesn't have xanthan gum, add 1 tsp of it. Most 1:1 blends already contain xanthan (or guar) gum.

Two hundred grams of flour is equivalent to 1¼ cups + 2 tbsp of Bob's Red Mill 1:1 Gluten-Free Flour Blend.

If cutting pasta by hand, flatten the dough into long, flat sheets. Roll into sheets and then cut the rolls into even strips.

Tip! Don't feel like making homemade pasta? Store-bought gluten-free pasta has come a long way and will make this dish easy-peasy!

Flavorful Baked Blackened Salmon

Salmon offers a plethora of healthy omega-3 fats, making it a health-packed meal I love to make, eat and serve. This salmon recipe is easy and requires just a few simple ingredients, many I suspect you already have on hand in your pantry.

Serve this dish with a baked potato, crispy sweet potato fries, roasted asparagus or steamed broccoli.

Prep Time: 5 minutes
Cook Time: 10-15 minutes
Yields: 4 servings
Equipment: None

4 salmon filets (about 1.5 lbs)
1 tsp avocado or vegetable oil
2 tsp paprika
2 tsp dried Italian seasoning
½ tsp garlic powder
½ tsp kosher salt
¼ tsp cayenne pepper
4 lemon wedges

Preheat oven to 400° F. Line a baking sheet with parchment paper. Add salmon filets to the parchment paper. Brush the top and sides of each filet with oil. Set aside.

Combine paprika, dried Italian seasoning, garlic, salt, and pepper in a small bowl, then evenly coat the seasonings over the fish's top and sides.

Bake fish for 12-14 minutes until salmon is cooked through. Top with a squeeze of lemon juice and serve immediately.

SAVORY MUSHROOM AND PEA RISOTTO

Rice is a staple grain for gluten-free eaters, and I love learning new ways to enjoy it. This light risotto recipe tastes amazing and can be a comforting side dish or the main entree. Most risottos are loaded with heavy creams, butter and cheese, but mine is dairy-free and light. Be sure to use Arborio rice. It's a short-grained rice with a high starch content. It offers up a creamy texture consistent with risotto.

Prep Time: 10 minutes
Cook Time: 45 minutes
Yield: 8 servings
Equipment: Small pot and large pan

5 ¾ cups chicken or vegetable broth
1 tbsp avocado or vegetable oil
1 large onion (about 2 cups), finely chopped
12 ounces portabella mushrooms, roughly chopped
2 garlic cloves, finely chopped
1 tsp kosher salt
Fresh ground pepper, to taste
1 ½ cups Arborio rice
⅔ cup dry white wine
¾ cup frozen peas, thawed

In a small pot, bring the broth to a rolling boil.

Heat oil over medium high heat in a large pan, then add onions and cook until softened, about 4-5 minutes. Add mushrooms and garlic and cook for another 10 minutes until mushrooms are cooked through and all juices have boiled off.

Add salt, pepper and rice and stir for another minute, then add white wine and cook until all the liquid is absorbed. Reduce heat to medium and add 1 cup of the hot broth to the rice mixture at a time. Cook until the liquid is absorbed, stirring continuously, for about 3 minutes. Continue to add liquid to mixture 1 cup at a time until the liquid is absorbed, stirring continuously, until all the liquid is absorbed into the rice mixture and the rice is creamy and soft (albeit slightly al dente), about 15-20 minutes. Reduce heat to low and gently fold in peas. Serve immediately.

COMFORTING CARROT AND WALNUT SOUP

There's nothing quite like fresh carrot soup that brings a smile to my face and warms my body and soul. My version of carrot soup, inspired by my friend Sarah Lehrfield, is extra special because not only does it contain hearty vegetables, but also it provides healthy fats thanks to the addition of walnuts.

Have you ever noticed how a walnut looks like a brain, and, coincidentally, contains plenty of brain-boosting omega-3 fatty acids. Eat - err - drink up!

Prep Time: 20 minutes
Cook Time: 55 minutes
Yield: 8-10 servings
Equipment: Handheld immersion blender, high-speed blender or food processor, large stock pot

2 tbsp avocado or vegetable oil
2 lbs fresh organic carrots, peeled and sliced into two-inch pieces
1 yellow onion, cut into large chunks
½ cup walnuts, shelled
6 cups chicken or vegetable broth
Kosher salt, to taste
Fresh ground pepper, to taste

Heat oil in a large stockpot over medium-high heat. Once oil is hot, add carrots and onion. Cover and cook for 10 minutes, stirring occasionally. Uncover, and add walnuts, broth, and salt and pepper to the pan and bring mixture to a boil. Once boiling, cover and reduce heat to a low simmer. Simmer for 45-60 minutes until carrots are soft when you press on them.

Blend the mixture into a smooth soup using your handheld immersion blender, a high-speed blender or food processor, working in batches. Serve immediately.

Tip! Serve with my Easy From-Scratch Sandwich Bread.

EASY SLOW COOKER MEATBALLS AND SPAGHETTI SQUASH

You're going to love my spin on this classic meal, which is a home-run dish and perfect for busy nights when I don't have time to cook. I cook the squash right on top of the meatballs inside the slow cooker, ensuring that I don't have to cook anything once I've added all the ingredients into the slow cooker.

You can cook the meatballs in a homemade sauce, or do what I do and use a jarred spaghetti sauce instead. Season the sauce and meatballs as you wish (it's truly a no-fail recipe). If anyone doesn't like the spaghetti squash, prepare a side of brown rice pasta for squash nay-sayers.

Prep Time: 15 minutes
Cook Time: 4 hours
Yield: 4 servings
Equipment: Slow cooker

1 25-ounce jar gluten-free marinara sauce*
1-1.25 lbs ground turkey
¼ cup brown rice flour (or gluten-free breadcrumbs)
1 large egg
1 tbsp olive oil
1 tsp garlic powder
1 tsp onion powder
1 tsp dried Italian seasoning
1 tsp kosher salt
¼ tsp fresh ground black pepper
1 spaghetti squash (medium)

Add sauce to the slow cooker and set aside.

Combine turkey, flour, egg, oil, and seasonings in a large bowl. Shape into about 8 evenly-sized meatballs and place each ball in the sauce until fully immersed.

Carefully slice spaghetti squash in half length-wise and remove seeds. Gently place squash on top of meatballs, cover the slow cooker, and set to cook on high for 4 hours.

Before serving, remove squash from the slow cooker with tongs and allow it to cool for about five minutes. Use your fork to scrape the squash flesh from the skin.

Divide squash, meatballs and sauce onto four plates and enjoy. Top with fresh basil or parmesan cheese (optional).

Notes:

   *I love using spicy marinara sauce. It adds so much bonus flavor to the mix. Mezzetta or Jersey Tomato make spicy marinara sauces that are free from gluten.

Favorite Simple Snacks

Whenever you get a hankering for a snack, try one of these 5 healthy, hunger-busting snack recipes.

Apple Butter Sandwiches

1 apple, cored and sliced
2-3 tbsp nut butter (almond butter, cashew butter, peanut butter, etc.)
1 tbsp mini chocolate chips

Slather each apple slice with nut butter, then top with a sprinkle of mini chocolate chips.

Avocado and Lime

½ avocado, pitted and removed from peel
1 lime wedge
¼ tsp kosher salt, Everything Bagel seasoning, or chili lime seasoning

Squeeze lime over avocado and sprinkle with kosher salt or seasoning of choice.

PB and Jam Rice Cake

1 rice cake
1 tbsp nut butter (almond butter, cashew butter, peanut butter, etc.)
1 tbsp jam or jelly of choice

Top rice cake with a layer of nut butter and jam. Enjoy immediately.

Vegetable Sticks with Guacamole

1 avocado, ripe
1 tsp red onion, finely chopped
1 tsp cilantro, finely chopped
Kosher salt, to taste
1-2 lime wedges
Sliced carrots, celery, cucumbers, and/or jicama

Mash avocado flesh in a bowl with a fork. Add red onion and cilantro and mix. Add salt and lime, to taste.

Serve with a melody of sliced vegetables or tortilla chips.

No-Bake Peanut Butter Bars

These no-bake peanut butter bars are perfect when you need a boost of on-the-go energy. Make these bars ahead of time and store them in your fridge for up to a week.

Prep Time: 10 minutes
Yield: 15 bars
Equipment: 8x8 baking dish

1½ cup gluten-free rolled oats
½ cup ground flaxseed
¼ cup protein powder
½ cup raisins or dried cranberries
½ cup + 1 tbsp mini chocolate chips, divided
½ tsp ground cinnamon
½ tsp kosher salt
1 cup natural peanut butter or almond butter
½ cup honey

Cover an 8×8-inch baking dish with parchment paper. Set aside.

In a large bowl, stir together oats, flaxseed meal, protein powder, dried cranberries, ½ cup of the mini chocolate chips, ground cinnamon, and kosher salt. Add peanut butter and honey to the mixture and stir until evenly combined. The mixture will be dry at first but will come together as the peanut butter and honey become more spread out. If extra moisture is needed to hold the mixture together, add more peanut butter.

Add the mixture to the prepared baking dish, and then press the mixture into a flat layer by hand. Sprinkle remaining 1 tablespoon of mini chocolate chips over the top and slightly press them into the mixture so they stick.

Chill mixture in the refrigerator to allow it to set for at least 1 hour before slicing into bars. Store bars in the fridge to keep cool.

FAVORITE BREADS, CAKES AND COOKIES

EASY FROM-SCRATCH SANDWICH BREAD

There are plenty of gluten-free store-bought breads available on the market today, but sometimes you crave homemade bread… and when you do, I've got you covered. This quick and easy sandwich bread is made with pantry staples, a 1:1 gluten-free flour blend, and just a few other simple ingredients.

Prep Time: 10 minutes
Cook Time: 38 minutes
Yield: About 18 slices
Equipment: Standing mixer, 8.5" x 4.5" loaf pan

3 cups Bob's Red Mill 1:1 Gluten-Free Flour blend (430 grams)
2 tbsp light brown sugar
2 tsp instant yeast, equivalent to 1 packet
2 tsp kosher salt
1 cup warm milk or dairy-free milk
1 tbsp raw honey
4 tbsp soft butter or vegan butter
3 large eggs

Combine flour, brown sugar, yeast, and salt in the bowl of your standing mixer and slowly mix all ingredients on low speed using paddle attachment. Drizzle in milk, then add honey and butter and continue to mix well.

Turn mixer to medium speed and add each egg, one at a time until incorporated. Once all the eggs are added, mix for another minute until dough is well combined. The batter will be sticky and soft (not like normal bread dough).

Add dough to a greased loaf pan, cover with plastic wrap, and allow it to rise for 90-120 minutes in a warm spot in your house.

Preheat oven to 350° F. When the oven comes to temperature, bake bread for 38-40 minutes until the top is slightly browned and the dough is cooked through. Place bread on a wire rack to cool completely.

Once cooled, use a serrated bread knife to cut bread into slices. The bread tastes fantastic toasted and lasts for several days when sealed in plastic wrap.

IRRESISTIBLY MOIST BANANA BREAD

It's time to turn those sad, spotted bananas into a happy and sweet banana bread. This recipe is so easy and fun to make. My son loves making banana bread (it's become his specialty) and this is his go-to recipe. The bread is sweet and chewy, and offers that doughy mouth appeal you might miss now that you can't eat gluten. Remember, the riper the bananas, the sweeter the bread. Adjust sugar amount accordingly.

Prep Time: 10 minutes
Cook Time: 50 minutes
Yield: 1 loaf or approximately 10 slices
Equipment: Standing mixer, 8.5" x 4.5" loaf pan

1½ cups of Bob's Red Mill 1:1 Gluten-Free Flour Blend
1 tsp baking soda
1 tsp kosher salt
½ tsp cinnamon
½ cup butter, softened
½ cup granulated sugar
2 large eggs
3 ripe bananas, mashed
½ tsp vanilla extract
½ cup chopped walnuts, raisins or chocolate chips (optional)

Preheat oven to 350° F and lightly grease your loaf pan. Set aside.

In a large bowl, sift together flour, baking soda, salt, and cinnamon. Set aside.

Using your mixer, cream butter and sugar together, then add eggs, bananas and vanilla and continue to mix on medium speed until all wet ingredients are combined. Add the flour mixture slowly into the wet mixture and mix on low until well combined. Fold in walnuts, raisins, or chocolate chips (optional) using your spatula, then pour batter into a lightly greased loaf pan.

Bake for 50 minutes until the top lightly browns and a toothpick inserted into the center comes out clean.

Tip! Don't have bananas? Substitute ½ cup of canned pumpkin or applesauce per banana and turn your banana bread into a whole new delicious treat!

Heavenly Almond Flour Lemon Crinkle Cookies

These lemon crinkle cookies taste like soft, lemon-drop candy. I make them for my friends who eat grain free and low-carb. Almond flour is made from ground, blanched almonds and is higher in fat, protein, and fiber than white refined flour. Because of almond flour's high fat content, these cookies are moist and chewy - yum!

Prep Time: 10 minutes
Cook Time: 25 minutes
Yields: 20 cookies
Equipment: Standing or handheld mixer

2 cups blanched almond flour
1 cup sugar
Pinch of salt
Zest of 1 lemon
2 large egg whites, room temperature
1 tsp fresh squeezed lemon juice
1/4 cup powdered sugar (for rolling)

Preheat oven to 350º F. Line a baking sheet with parchment paper and set it aside.

In a medium mixing bowl, combine almond flour, sugar, salt and lemon zest. Mix together and set aside.

Using your standing or handheld mixer, beat egg whites until soft peaks form, then fold in lemon juice and almond flour mixture into the egg whites, by hand, until well combined.

Using lightly wet hands, roll dough into 1.5-inch balls and set aside. Dry hands and then roll each ball in powdered sugar. Place each ball on a prepared baking sheet about 2 inches apart.

Bake for 15-17 minutes or until tops start to crack and bottoms are slightly browned. Cool completely before serving. These cookies store well and taste amazing for several days after baking.

No-Fail Chocolate Chip Applesauce Cake

This is my absolute favorite gluten-free chocolate dessert recipe, and it's inspired by a recipe first introduced to our family by my husband's grandmother, Bubu. I loved making and eating this cake in my pre-celiac years, and I thought I would never get to enjoy it again when I was diagnosed with celiac disease. However, thanks to the advent of 1:1 gluten-free flours, I was able to make this cake and eat it too!

Prep Time: 20 minutes
Bake Time: 35 minutes
Yields: 16 servings
Equipment: 9" x 13" baking dish

Cake:

½ cup butter, equal to 1 stick
1½ cups sugar
2 large eggs
2½ cups unsweetened applesauce
1 tsp vanilla
½ tsp cinnamon
2 cups Bob's Red Mill 1:1 Gluten-Free Flour Blend (about 280 grams)
½ tsp salt
1½ tsp baking soda
2 heaping tbsp cocoa

Topping:

2 cups chocolate chips
5 tbsp brown sugar

Preheat oven to 350° F. Line the baking dish with foil, spray with cooking spray, and set aside.

In a mixer, cream together butter and sugar. Add eggs, applesauce, vanilla, and cinnamon and mix until well combined.

In a separate bowl, sift together flour, salt, baking soda and cocoa, then add the flour mixture slowly to the wet mixture, mixing on low and scraping sides occasionally to ensure all ingredients are well combined. Transfer mixture to greased baking pan.

Generously sprinkle chocolate chips and brown sugar over the batter until cake is well covered, and place the baking pan in the oven for 35-40 minutes until a toothpick comes out clean when inserted into the center.

DELICIOUS SOOTHING DRINKS AND BLENDS

Juicing can help you rest your digestive system and flood your body with the essential nutrients it has been missing for much too long.

When making a juice recipe of your own, follow this simple recipe:

- 1 part leafy green vegetable (i.e. kale, spinach, Swiss chard)
- 1 part juicy vegetable (i.e. celery, cucumber, beet, carrots, peppers)
- 1 part juicy fruit (i.e. mango, pineapple, apple, pear, peeled orange)
- Flavor enhancements (i.e. squeeze of lemon, ginger, mint leaves)

The key to a good juice is to have two portions of vegetables to one portion of fruit. The fruit simply sweetens the juice to help it go down more smoothly. Use less fruit and work your way up, creating juices with more vegetables than fruit.

You can find additional juice recipes at goodforyouglutenfree.com.

Jenny's Go-To Green Juice

This refreshing green juice will flood your body with a slew of vitamins and minerals, coating your insides with healthy green goodness. To add a touch of sweetness, add a chunk of pineapple (my favorite fruit to juice). Use more pineapple if you like it sweeter, less once you become accustomed to drinking green juice. This drink goes down smoothly and effortlessly.

Prep Time: 5 minutes
Yield: 1 8-ounce serving
Equipment: Juicer

3-4 stalks of fresh kale (leaf and stem intact)
2 celery stalks
1/3 English cucumber
1 large chunk of fresh pineapple (3-4 large cubes)
½ small lemon, peeled with white pith intact (optional)
1 inch peeled fresh ginger

Run each ingredient through your juicer one at a time, applying firm pressure, until each item is fully processed. The celery and cucumber can be used to help push through the leafy greens and smaller ingredients. Enjoy immediately.

TURMERIC TONIC ORANGE JUICE

Turmeric helps fight inflammation and is a potent antioxidant. Use fresh turmeric root in this recipe to boost your immune system and tame inflammation naturally. You can find turmeric root at most grocery stores. It looks a lot like ginger root, except its flesh is bright orange in color.

Prep Time: 5 minutes
Yield: 1 8-ounce serving
Equipment: Juicer

3 large chunks of cantaloupe, peeled and seeded
1/2 grapefruit or orange, peeled with white pith intact
1/4 lemon, peeled
1/2 inch fresh ginger root, peeled
1/2 inch fresh turmeric root, peeled

Wash and prepare all ingredients, then run each ingredient through your juicer, one-by-one. Serve immediately.

SEA SALT GREEN SMOOTHIE

This refreshing smoothie blends together some of my favorite vegetables and fruits with a touch of sea salt to add flavor and trace minerals to your smoothie.

Prep Time: 2 minutes
Yield: 1 8-ounce serving
Equipment: High-speed blender

4 celery stalks
Large bunch of spinach
3/4 cup frozen pineapple
1 cup filtered water
Dash of sea salt
Dash of cayenne pepper

Wash and prepare all ingredients. Add all ingredients to your high-speed blender and blend until smooth, about 45-60 seconds. Serve immediately.

ACKNOWLEDGEMENTS

Writing a book is fulfilling a lifelong dream. I am filled with a variety of emotions as this book, which I've been working on for years, is finally coming to life. It's hard to put myself out there and share my truths with all of you. Thank you for allowing me the safe space to do it via my blog, Good For You Gluten Free, and now through this book.

I'd like to acknowledge a few people who have been a part of my journey:

First, I am truly grateful for you, my loyal readers and followers. You have been with me through the ups and downs, and have inspired me to persevere.

Thank you to my supportive husband, Darren. You know exactly how to motivate me to keep going and push through the difficult moments. You are the best advisor, too. Thank you for loving me unconditionally, celiac disease and all.

Thank you to my children, Benjamin and Sydney, for always having my back and making sure your mom is always included when food is a part of the plan.

Thank you to my parents and in-laws for always loving and supporting me, and for making sure there is always something gluten free for me to eat at family get-togethers.

Thank you to my friend, Andrea Ruccolo, for waking me up and teaching me how to heal my body from the inside out.

Thank you to Kathy Passerine for your encouragement and critical editing eye. Your generosity and willingness to jump in and help means so much. I don't know how I'll ever repay you for your kindness.

Thank you to Beatie Deutsch, Dana Vollmer, Shannon Ford, Patrick Strompoli, and Nichole Thomas for saying "yes" to sharing your stories and struggles with me – and the gluten-free community – in the pages of this book.

Thank you to Dr. Tom O'Bryan, for shedding light on the seriousness of all gluten disorders, inspiring a community that extends well beyond celiac disease, and for believing in me, and this project, by lending your name and words to the beautiful Foreword of this book.

Thank you to Stephanie Chandler and my publishing family at Authority Publishing. I appreciate your guidance, advice, and candor.

Finally, thank you to God, for helping me to find meaning in my challenges. I am truly blessed.

ENDNOTES

1   De Santis MA, Kosik O, Passmore D, Flagella Z, Shewry PR, Lovegrove A. Comparison of the dietary fibre composition of old and modern durum wheat (Triticum turgidum spp. durum) genotypes. *Food Chem.* 2018;244:304-310. doi:10.1016/j.foodchem.2017.09.143

2   Bressan P, Kramer P. Bread and Other Edible Agents of Mental Disease. *Front Hum Neurosci.* 2016;10:130. Published 2016 Mar 29. doi:10.3389/fnhum.2016.00130

3   Teshima R. *Yakugaku Zasshi.* 2014;134(1):33-38. doi:10.1248/yakushi.13-00209-2

4   Tranquet O, Larré C, Denery-Papini S. Allergic reactions to hydrolysed wheat proteins: clinical aspects and molecular structures of the allergens involved. *Crit Rev Food Sci Nutr.* 2020;60(1):147-156. doi:10.1080/10408398.2018.1516622

5   Celiac Disease Foundation, "20 Things You Might Not Know about Celiac Disease." August 20, 2016.

6   Giacomo Caio, Umberto Volta, Anna Sapone, Daniel A. Leffler, Roberto De Giorgio, Carlo Catassi & Alessio Fasano, "Celiac disease: a comprehensive current review." BMC Medicine. 23 July 2019. 17:142

7   University of Chicago Celiac Disease Center Frequently Asked Questions https://www.cureceliacdisease.org/faq/how-many-people-in-the-united-states-have-celiac-disease/

8   Lauret E, Rodrigo L. Celiac disease and autoimmune-associated conditions. Biomed Res Int. 2013;2013:127589. doi:10.1155/2013/127589. Epub 2013 Jul 24. PMID: 23984314; PMCID: PMC3741914.

9   Environmental Research, "Persistent organic pollutant exposure and celiac disease: A pilot study," 11 May 2020. Abigail Gaylord Leonardo Trasande Krunthachalam Kannan Kristen M. Thomas Sunmi Leef Mengling Liu, Jeremiah Levine.

10 Canadian Society of Intestinal Research. Celiac Disease: Still Vastly Under-Diagnosed | Gastrointestinal Society by Shelley Case.

11 Ann Cranney, Marion Zarkadas, Ian D. Graham, J. Decker Butzner, Mohsin Rashid, Ralph Warren, Mavis Molloy, Shelley Case, Vernon Burrows, Connie Switzer, "Canadian Celiac Health Survey." *Digestive Diseases and Sciences*. 13 November 2005.

12 O'Bryan, Dr. Tom, "You Can Fix Your Brain." (Rodale 2018), pg 136.

13 Di Sabatino A, Volta U, Salvatore C, et al. Small Amounts of Gluten in Subjects With Suspected Nonceliac Gluten Sensitivity: A Randomized, Double-Blind, Placebo-Controlled, Cross-Over Trial. Clin Gastroenterol Hepatol. 2015;13(9):1604-12.e3. doi:10.1016/j.cgh.2015.01.029

14 Hollon J, Puppa EL, Greenwald B, Goldberg E, Guerrerio A, Fasano A. Effect of gliadin on permeability of intestinal biopsy explants from celiac disease patients and patients with non-celiac gluten sensitivity. *Nutrients*. 2015;7(3):1565-1576. Published 2015 Feb 27.

15 https://www.ncbi.nlm.nih.gov/pubmed/25734566

16 Bryant-Erdmann, Stephanie, "Human Wheat Consumption Sets New Record," US Wheat Associates. 14 November 2018.

17 Davis, Dr. William, "Wheat Belly." (Rodale 2011), pg 6.

18 Wheat Belly pg 13

19 Wheat Belly pg 14

20 Wheat Belly pg 18

21 Wheat Belly pg 24

22 Wheat Belly pg 24

23 Wheat Belly pgs 25-26

24 Liu E, Dong F, Barón AE, et al. High Incidence of Celiac Disease in a Long-term Study of Adolescents With Susceptibility Genotypes. Gastroenterology. 2017;152(6):1329-1336.e1. doi:10.1053/j.gastro.2017.02.002

25 "Once is Enough: A Guide to Preventing Future Fractures." National Institute of Arthritis and Musculoskeletal and Skin Disease

26   "Li K, Wang XF, Li DY, et al. The good, the bad, and the ugly of calcium supplementation: a review of calcium intake on human health. Clin Interv Aging. 2018;13:2443-2452. Published 2018 Nov 28.

27   Dryden, Jim. "Osteoporosis patients should be screened for celiac disease, study says." 28 February 2005.

28   Cojocaru M, Cojocaru IM, Silosi I. Multiple autoimmune syndrome. *Maedica (Buchar)*. 2010;5(2):132-134.

29   "Dermatitis Herpetiformis (For Health Care Professionals)," The National Institute of Diabetes and Digestive and Kidney Diseases Health Information Center. February 2014. https://www.niddk.nih.gov/health-information/professionals/clinical-tools-patient-management/digestive-diseases/dermatitis-herpetiformis

30   Hansen D, Bennedbaek FN, Hansen LK, et al. High prevalence of coeliac disease in Danish children with type I diabetes mellitus. *Acta Paediatr*. 2001;90(11):1238-1243.

31   "Inflammatory Bowel Disease, Celiac Are Linked: Review," by Robert Preidt. US News & World Report, 1 June 2020.

32   Perlmutter, Dr. David, "Grain Brain," (Little, Brown, and Company 2013) pg 32

33   Grain Brain pg 60

34   Cigic L, Galic T, Kero D, et al. The prevalence of celiac disease in patients with geographic tongue. J Oral Pathol Med. 2016;45(10):791-796. doi:10.1111/jop.12450

35   WebMD, "Cold Sores." https://www.webmd.com/skin-problems-and-treatments/understanding-cold-sores-basics#1

36   Seehusen DA. Comparative Accuracy of Diagnostic Tests for Celiac Disease. *Am Fam Physician*. 2017;95(11):726-728.

37   You Can Fix Your Brain pg 45

38   University of Chicago Celiac Disease Center Frequently Asked Questions, http://www.cureceliacdisease.org/faq/are-raised-dgp-igg-levels-an-early-sign-of-celiac-disease/

39   The Conundrum of Gluten Sensitivity by Dr. Tom O'Bryan. November 2014.

40   Genetic and Rare Diseases Information Center, "Celiac Disease." https://rarediseases.info.nih.gov/diseases/11998/celiac-disease/cases/43805

41 Beyond Celiac, "The Gluten Challenge." https://www.beyondceliac. org/celiac-disease/the-gluten-challenge/

42 Kim H, Patel KG, Orosz E, et al. Time Trends in the Prevalence of Celiac Disease and Gluten-Free Diet in the US Population: Results From the National Health and Nutrition Examination Surveys 2009-2014. JAMA Intern Med. 2016;176(11):1716–1717. doi:10.1001/jamainternmed.2016.5254

43 "Is Maltodextrin Gluten Free?" *Beyond Celiac* website. https://www. beyondceliac.org/gluten-free-diet/is-it-gluten-free/maltodextrin/

44 "Vinegar: When Is It Gluten Free?" by Trishia Thompson, *Diet.com*. 2 June 2009.

45 "What Alcohol Is Gluten Free?" University of Chicago School of Medicine. 13 December 2018. https://www.uchicagomedicine.org/ forefront/gastrointestinal-articles/is-alcohol-gluten-free

46 Niaz K, Zaplatic E, Spoor J. Extensive use of monosodium glutamate: A threat to public health?. *EXCLI J*. 2018;17:273-278. Published 2018 Mar 19. doi:10.17179/excli2018-1092

47 NASSCD Releases Summary Statement on Oats, Celiac Disease Foundation. 25 April 2016.

48 Lerner, Benjamin A. MD1; Phan Vo, Lynn T. BA2; Yates, Shireen MBA3; Rundle, Andrew G. DrPH2; Green, Peter H.R. MD1; Lebwohl, Benjamin MD, MS1,2 Detection of Gluten in Gluten-Free Labeled Restaurant Food, American Journal of Gastroenterology: May 2019 - Volume 114 - Issue 5 - p 792-797 doi: 10.14309/ ajg.0000000000000202

49 Enforcing the ADA: A Status Report from the Department of Justice, July-September 2004. U.S. Department of Justice, Civil Rights Division, Disability Rights Section.

50 "An integrated, accurate, rapid, and economical handheld consumer gluten detector," by Jingqing Zhanga, Steven Barbosa, Portela Joseph, Benjamin Horrella, Alex Leunga, Dane Rene Weitmanna, John Boguslaw Artiucha, Stephen Michael Wilsona, Monica Cipriania, Lyndsie Katherine Slakey, Aquanette Michele Burta, Francisco Javier Dias Lourenco, Marc Stephen Spinalia, Jonathan Robert Ward AlimSeit-Nebib Scott Erik Sundvora, Shireen Natasha Yates. Food Chemistry. Volume 275, 1 March 2019, Pages 446-456.

51 "Inactive" ingredients in oral medications," by Daniel Reker, Steven M. Blum, Christoph Steiger, Kevin E. Anger, Jamie M. Sommer, John Fanikos, Giovanni Traverso. *Science Translational Medicine*. 13 Mar 2019

52 "Gluten in Drug Products and Associated Labeling Recommendations Guidance for Industry," by U.S. Department of Health and Human Services Food and Drug Administration. December 2017

53 Email to Johnson & Johnson Customer Care Center dated June 9, 2019, REF# 001038288.

54 Wheat Belly pg 43

55 "Wheat is an Opiate," by Dr. William Davis. WheatBellyBlog, 17 April 2012 https://www.wheatbellyblog.com/2012/04/wheat-is-an-opiate/

56 Wheat Belly pg 45

57 You Can Fix Your Brain pg 164

58 Wheat Belly pg 53

59 Wheat Belly pg 66

60 Carroccio A, D'Alcamo A, Cavataio F, et al. High Proportions of People With Nonceliac Wheat Sensitivity Have Autoimmune Disease or Antinuclear Antibodies. *Gastroenterology*. 2015;149(3):596-603. e1. doi:10.1053/j.gastro.2015.05.040

61 Grain Brain pg 50

62 Mucosal Healing and Risk for Lymphoproliferative Malignancy in Celiac Disease, by Benjamin Lebwohl, Fredrik Granath, Anders Ekbom, Karin E. Smedby, Joseph A. Murray, Alfred I. Neugut, Peter H.R. Green, and Jonas F. Ludvigsson. *Annals of Internal Medicine*. 2013 159:3, 169-175.

63 Rubio-Tapia A, Kyle RA, Kaplan EL, et al. Increased prevalence and mortality in undiagnosed celiac disease. *Gastroenterology*. 2009;137(1):88-93. doi:10.1053/j.gastro.2009.03.059

64 West J, Logan RF, Smith CJ, Hubbard RB, Card TR. Malignancy and mortality in people with coeliac disease: population based cohort study. *BMJ*. 2004;329(7468):716-719. doi:10.1136/bmj.38169.486701.7C

65 Askling J, Linet M, Gridley G, Halstensen TS, Ekström K, Ekbom A. Cancer incidence in a population-based cohort of

individuals hospitalized with celiac disease or dermatitis herpeti-formis. *Gastroenterology*. 2002;123(5):1428-1435. doi:10.1053/gast.2002.36585

[66] Lebwohl B, Green PHR, Söderling J, Roelstraete B, Ludvigsson JF. Association Between Celiac Disease and Mortality Risk in a Swedish Population. *JAMA*. 2020;323(13):1277–1285. doi:10.1001/jama.2020.1943

[67] "Mortality in patients with coeliac disease and their relatives: a cohort study," by Dr Prof Giovanni Corrao, PhD, Prof Gino Roberto Corazza, MD, Vincenzo Bagnardi, PhD, Giovanna Brusco, MD, Carolina Ciacci, MD, Mario Cottone, MD, et al. *The Lancet*. August 04, 2001 DOI:https://doi.org/10.1016/S0140-6736(01)05554-4

[68] Ludvigsson JF, Montgomery SM, Ekbom A, Brandt L, Granath F. Small-intestinal histopathology and mortality risk in celiac disease. *JAMA*. 2009;302(11):1171-1178. doi:10.1001/jama.2009.1320

[69] O'Bryan, Dr. Tom, "The Autoimmune Fix." (Rodale 2016) pg 29

[70] "Doctors Once Thought Bananas Cured Celiac Disease. They Saved Kids' Lives — At A Cost," by Jill Neimark. NPR.org 24 March 2017.

[71] "Overcoming Motherhood Imposter Syndrome. Casey Wilson learned to trust her parenting instincts after her son received a surprise diagnosis." by Casey Wilson. *The New York Times*. 15 April 2020.

[72] Eger, Dr. Edith, "The Choice: Embrace the Impossible." (Scribner 2017).

[73] Shah S, Akbari M, Vanga R, et al. Patient perception of treatment burden is high in celiac disease compared with other common conditions. *Am J Gastroenterol*. 2014;109(9):1304-1311. doi:10.1038/ajg.2014.29

[74] Häuser W, Janke KH, Klump B, Gregor M, Hinz A. Anxiety and depression in adult patients with celiac disease on a gluten-free diet. *World J Gastroenterol*. 2010;16(22):2780-2787. doi:10.3748/wjg.v16.i22.2780

[75] Penn State. "Women with celiac disease suffer from depression, disordered eating, study finds," *Science Daily*. 27 December 2011

[76] Eger, Dr. Edith, "The Choice: Embrace the Impossible." (Scribner 2017).

77   "Partner Burden: A Common Entity in Celiac Disease," by Abhik
Roy, Maria Minaya, Milka Monegro, Jude Fleming, Reuben K.
Wong, Suzanne Lewis, Benjamin Lebwohl, and Peter H. R. Green.
Digestive Diseases and Sciences. 17 April 2016

78   "Going gluten-free could leave you single because almost half of
people would judge someone on the diet as 'selfish, demanding
and difficult to please'," by Alexandra Thompson. Daily Mail. 25
September 2018

79   Celiac Disease Facts and Figures, The University of Chicago School
of Medicine.

80   Wheat Belly pg 65

81   Lanzini A, Lanzarotto F, Villanacci V, et al. Complete recovery
of intestinal mucosa occurs very rarely in adult coeliac patients
despite adherence to gluten-free diet. *Aliment Pharmacol Ther.*
2009;29(12):1299-1308. doi:10.1111/j.1365-2036.2009.03992.

82   "How Much Do Doctors Learn About Nutrition? The answer: It
may not be enough – but it's not their fault," by Stacey Colino. *U.S.
News and World Report.* 7 December 2016.

83   Ibid

84   Radical Remission. Surviving Cancer Against All Odds by Kelly A.
Turner, Ph.D.

85   "Your gut is directly connected to your brain, by a newly discovered
neuron circuit," By Emily Underwood. *Science.* 20 September 2018.

86   Qin J, Li R, Raes J, et al. A human gut microbial gene catalogue estab-
lished by metagenomic sequencing. *Nature.* 2010;464(7285):59-65.
doi:10.1038/nature08821

87   Grain Brain pg 8

88   Fast Facts about The Human Microbiome, The Center for Ecogenetics
and Environmental Health, University of Washington, 1/2014.

89   de Sousa Moraes LF, Grzeskowiak LM, de Sales Teixeira TF, Gouveia
Peluzio Mdo C. Intestinal microbiota and probiotics in celiac
disease. *Clin Microbiol Rev.* 2014;27(3):482-489. doi:10.1128/
CMR.00106-13

90   "Digestion of Intact Gluten Proteins by Bifidobacterium Species:
Reduction of Cytotoxicity and Proinflammatory Responses," by
Natália Ellen Castilho de Almeida, Franciele Grego Esteves, José

Roberto Aparecido dos Santos-Pinto, Carla Peres de Paula, etc. al. Journal of Agriculture Food Chemistry, 20 March 2020.

91   Cristofori F, Indrio F, Miniello VL, De Angelis M, Francavilla R. Probiotics in Celiac Disease. *Nutrients*. 2018;10(12):1824. Published 2018 Nov 23. doi:10.3390/nu10121824

92   Corouge M, Loridant S, Fradin C, et al. Humoral immunity links Candida albicans infection and celiac disease. *PLoS One*. 2015;10(3):e0121776. Published 2015 Mar 20. doi:10.1371/journal.pone.0121776

93   Harnett J, Myers SP, Rolfe M. Significantly higher faecal counts of the yeasts *candida* and *saccharomyces* identified in people with coeliac disease. *Gut Pathog*. 2017;9:26. Published 2017 May 5. doi:10.1186/s13099-017-0173-1

94   Evans KE, Higham S, Smythe A, *et al*, Small bowel bacterial overgrowth in coeliac disease: a cause of presenting symptoms? *Gut* 2011; 60:A83-A84.

95   Dukowicz AC, Lacy BE, Levine GM. Small intestinal bacterial overgrowth: a comprehensive review. *Gastroenterol Hepatol (N Y)*. 2007;3(2):112-122.

96   Yang Q. Gain weight by "going diet?" Artificial sweeteners and the neurobiology of sugar cravings: Neuroscience 2010. *Yale J Biol Med*. 2010;83(2):101-108.

97   Grain Brain pg 104

98   "Glycemic index and firming kinetics of partially baked frozen gluten-free bread with sourdough," by Dubravka Novotni, Nikolina Čukelj, Bojana Smerdel, Martina Bituh, Filip Dujmić Duška. *Journal of Cereal Science*. Volume 55, Issue 2, March 2012, Pages 120-125.

99   "Americans Eat their Weight in Genetically Engineered Foods," by Renee Sharp. *AgMag*. 15 October 2012.

100   The Facts About Glyphosate, Part 1: How Do Wheat Growers Use Glyphosate by The National Wheat Foundation. https://wheatfoundation.org/the-truth-about-glyphosate-part-1-how-do-wheat-growers-use-glyphosate/

101   "How GMO Technology Saved the Papaya," by Elizabeth Held. International Food Information Council Foundation. 14 June 2016.

[102] Bezanson GS, MacInnis R, Potter G, Hughes T. Presence and potential for horizontal transfer of antibiotic resistance in oxidase-positive bacteria populating raw salad vegetables. Int J Food Microbiol. 2008;127(1–2):37–42.

[103] Genetic and Rare Diseases Information Center, https://rarediseases.info.nih.gov/diseases/11998/celiac-disease/cases/43805#ref_7161

[104] Changing Your Diet Can Make You Live Longer, by Alice Park. Time. 12 July 2017.

[105] Intermittent fasting: Surprising update - Harvard Health Blog by Monique Tello. *Harvard Health Blog*, 29 June 2018.

[106] Kim JA, Kim JY, Kang SW. Effects of the Dietary Detoxification Program on Serum γ-glutamyltransferase, Anthropometric Data and Metabolic Biomarkers in Adults. *J Lifestyle Med*. 2016;6(2):49-57. doi:10.15280/jlm.2016.6.2.49

[107] Wierdsma NJ, van Bokhorst-de van der Schueren MA, Berkenpas M, Mulder CJ, van Bodegraven AA. Vitamin and mineral deficiencies are highly prevalent in newly diagnosed celiac disease patients. *Nutrients*. 2013;5(10):3975-3992. Published 2013 Sep 30. doi:10.3390/nu5103975

[108] Nair R, Maseeh A. Vitamin D: The "sunshine" vitamin. *J Pharmacol Pharmacother*. 2012;3(2):118-126. doi:10.4103/0976-500X.95506

[109] Gubatan J, Moss AC. Vitamin D in inflammatory bowel disease: more than just a supplement. *Curr Opin Gastroenterol*. 2018;34(4):217-225. doi:10.1097/MOG.0000000000000449

[110] Dahele A, Ghosh S. Vitamin B12 deficiency in untreated celiac disease. *Am J Gastroenterol*. 2001;96(3):745-750. doi:10.1111/j.1572-0241.2001.03616.x

[111] Ibid

[112] "Thompson T. Folate, iron, and dietary fiber contents of the gluten-free diet. *J Am Diet Assoc*. 2000;100(11):1389-1396. doi:10.1016/S0002-8223(00)00386-2

[113] Calder PC. Omega-3 fatty acids and inflammatory processes. *Nutrients*. 2010;2(3):355-374. doi:10.3390/nu2030355

[114] Maroon JC, Bost JW. Omega-3 fatty acids (fish oil) as an anti-inflammatory: an alternative to nonsteroidal anti-inflammatory

drugs for discogenic pain. Surg Neurol. 2006;65(4):326-331. doi:10.1016/j.surneu.2005.10.023

[115] "If David Ludwig Is Right, Everything We Thought We Knew About Obesity—and Low-Fat Diets—Is Wrong," by Philip J. Hilts. *Boston Magazine.* 5 January 2016.

[116] "The U.S. Obesity Rate Now Tops 40%," by Gabby Galvin. *US News and World Report.* 27 February 2020.

[117] Kaplan M, Ates I, Yüksel M, et al. The Role of Oxidative Stress in the Etiopathogenesis of Gluten-sensitive Enteropathy Disease. *J Med Biochem.* 2017;36(3):243-250. Published 2017 Jul 14. doi:10.1515/jomb-2017-0017

[118] Kristjánsson G, Venge P, Hällgren R. Mucosal reactivity to cow's milk protein in coeliac disease. *Clin Exp Immunol.* 2007;147(3):449-455. doi:10.1111/j.1365-2249.2007.03298.

[119] Jacofsky D, Jacofsky EM, Jacofsky M. Understanding Antibody Testing for COVID-19. J Arthroplasty. 2020;35(7S):S74-S81. doi:10.1016/j.arth.2020.04.055

[120] Skodje GI, Sarna VK, Minelle IH, et al. Fructan, Rather Than Gluten, Induces Symptoms in Patients With Self-Reported Non-Celiac Gluten Sensitivity. *Gastroenterology.* 2018;154(3):529-539.e2. doi:10.1053/j.gastro.2017.10.040

[121] Brighten, Dr. Jolene, "Beyond the Pill." (HarperOne, 2019) pgs 106-107.

[122] International Society for Environmentally Acquired Illness About EAI page, https://iseai.org/about-eai/

[123] Ibid

[124] Gaylord A, Trasande L, Kannan K, et al. Persistent organic pollutant exposure and celiac disease: A pilot study. *Environ Res.* 2020;186:109439. doi:10.1016/j.envres.2020.109439

[125] Ciacci C, Siniscalchi M, Bucci C, Zingone F, Morra I, Iovino P. Life events and the onset of celiac disease from a patient's perspective. *Nutrients.* 2013;5(9):3388-3398. Published 2013 Aug 28. doi:10.3390/nu5093388

[126] University of California - Los Angeles. "Study shows how serotonin and a popular anti-depressant affect the gut's microbiota." ScienceDaily. ScienceDaily, 6 September 2019.

127 Stress Hormone Causes Epigenetic Changes, by National Institutes of Health. 27 September 2010.

128 Exercise and stress: Get moving to manage stress by Mayo Clinic Staff. 8 March 2018.

129 Refractory Celiac Disease - National Organization for Rare Disorders by Ciarán P. Kelly, MD

130 Rubio-Tapia A, Murray JA. Classification and management of refractory coeliac disease. *Gut.* 2010;59(4):547-557. doi:10.1136/gut.2009.195131

131 Nearly One in Two Americans Takes Prescription Drugs: Survey by Shelly Hagan. *Bloomberg.com.* 7 May 2019.

INDEX

Visit goodforyouglutenfree.com for more information and recipes.

"Healing is a matter of time, but it is sometimes also a matter of opportunity."

- Hippocrates